MW01231596

Air Fryer Cookbook On a Budget

Top 60 Air Fryer Recipes with Low Salt, Low Fat and Less Oil.

Amazingly Easy Recipes to Fry, Bake, Grill, and Roast with Your Air Fryer

Ronda Williams

Table of Contents

Introduction

What is Air Frying?

First, a quick explanation of what air frying is and isn't. They don't fry food at all. They are more like a self-contained convection oven than a deep fat fryer. Most units have one or more heating elements, along with a fan or two to circulate the hot air. These appliances quickly heat and circulate the hot air around and through the food in the tray. This cooking method takes advantage of the heat and the drying effect of the air to cook foods quickly, leaving them crisp and browned on the outside but still moist inside. While the results can be similar to using a deep fryer, they are not identical.

What Are The Pros And Cons Of An Air Fryer?

While the enthusiasm about these products may be a bit overblown, there are some solid benefits to using an air fryer, as well as some major downsides.

Pros of An Air Fryer

1. Healthier Meals

You do not need to use much (or any) oil in these appliances to get your food crispy and browned! Most users just spritz a little oil on the item and then proceed to the cooking cycle. The hot air takes advantage of the little bit of oil, and any excess oil just drains away from the food. This makes these devices ideal for making fresh and frozen fries, onion rings, mozzarella sticks, chicken wings, and nuggets. Unlike a traditional oven, air frying items are cooked faster and the excess oil doesn't soak into your food. So the claims that they use less oil and make healthier meals are true!

2. Quicker, More Efficient Cooking

Air fryers take just minutes to preheat, and most of the heat stays inside the appliance. Foods cook faster than in an oven or on a stovetop because this heat is not lost to the surrounding air. Even frozen foods are quickly cooked because the effect of the heat is intensified by the circulating air. These units are also more energy-efficient than an oven. Using a fryer will not heat your house in the summer, and the cost of the electricity used is just pennies. Since the cooking cycle is also shorter, you can see that using a fryer makes most cooking faster and more efficient than traditional appliances!

3. Versatility

You can use them to air fry, stir fry, reheat, bake, broil, roast, grill, steam, and even rotisserie in some models. Besides the fries and nuggets, you can make hot dogs and sausages, steak, chicken breasts or thighs, grilled sandwiches, stir-fried meats and veggies, roasted or steamed veggies, all kinds of fish and shrimp dishes, even cakes and desserts. If your unit is large enough, you can even bake a whole chicken or small turkey, or do a beef or pork roast. They are more than just a fryer!

4. Space-Saving

Most units are about the size of a coffee maker. Some models are small and super-compact, making them perfect for small kitchens, kitchenettes, dorm rooms, or RVs. An air fryer can replace an oven in a situation that lacks one and can be more useful than a toaster oven or steamer. If you use it frequently you will likely be happy to give it a home on your kitchen counter!

5. Easy To Use

Most fryers are designed to be easy to use. Just set the cooking temperature and time, put your food in the basket, and walk away. Of course, you will get better results if you shake your food once or twice during the cooking cycle, especially for things like fries, chips, wings, and nuggets. This ensures even browning and perfect results. Many air fryer enthusiasts have even taught their children to use them for making after school snacks or quick lunches!

Cons of An Air Fryer

1. Quality Issues

Air fryers are mostly made from plastic and inexpensive metal parts. They may or may not bear up after months or years of use. The heating elements, controls, and fans tend to go out eventually, and once they do your unit is useless. The metal cooking baskets and pans do not tend to last very long and often need to be replaced. Print on the dials or control panels can wear off. Even expensive units can have these issues, and some brands seem to have a lot of reported problems. These are not sturdy, long-lasting kitchen appliances overall.

2. Takes Up Space

Ok, I had "Space Saver" listed as a pro...how can it be a con as well? Easy! They do take up space, either on your counter or stored away in a cabinet. If you use it frequently this might not be a problem...but if you only drag it out to make the occasional batch of wings then the loss of space might not make it worth it to you. It depends on how and if you use it. Some units are fairly heavy as well, and might not be very easy to move around. They have the potential to be just another appliance you use a few times and then sell at a yard sale.

3. Not Ideal For Large Families

You will see some fryers advertised for "large families" but what does that mean? Most air fryers are best suited to making food for 1-4 people (depending on the capacity). There are very few that can handle making food for more than 4, and they often still require cooking in batches. For large families, a true convection air frying oven would probably be a better choice.

A medium-sized fryer with a capacity of 3.5 quarts can usually handle the main dish for two or a main and side dish for one. A large unit with a capacity of 5.8 quarts can handle the main dish like a whole chicken...which theoretically means enough to serve 4 people, as long as you cook the rest of the food in another appliance. So these are ideal for smaller families or single users, or a dorm or office snack maker.

4. Learning Curve

They ARE easy to use, but there is still a learning curve. Each unit has its peculiarities that you will have to figure out. They come with cooking guides and recipes, but those are more recommendations rather than firm instructions. It may take a few trials before you get the results that you want. Luckily the internet is filled with users who have shared their experiences, so finding tips is pretty easy.

5. Limitations

For all their versatility, air fryers have limitations as well. You are limited by the size and shape of the basket. Your frozen taquitos may not fit into some models, and you might be limited to a 6-inch pie pan in another. Food sometimes gets stuck to the cooking pans, meaning a more difficult clean-up for you. Even with accessories like elevated cooking racks and kabob skewers, you will still have to cook in batches or use another appliance if you are making food for multiple people. You also have to wait for the unit to cool off before cleaning and storing it away. For some people, these limitations might be too much to make an air fryer worth it.

Air Fryer Benefits

- An air fryer has many benefits to offer its customers.
- Low-fat meals
- Easy cleanup
- Uses hot-air circulation, the air fryer cooks your ingredients from all angles- with no oil needed.
- This ultimately produces healthier foods than most fryers and spares you from that unwanted aroma of fried foods in your home.
- To make sure you get the most out of your appliance, most fryers are accompanied by a recipe book to help you get started right away on your journey of fast, yet healthy meal preparations.

- Whether your favorite dish is french fries, muffins, chips, chicken tenders, or grilled vegetables, an air fryer can prepare it all.

Is an Air Fryer Useful?

At the tip of your fingers, you can have an appliance that specializes in making delicious, healthy meals that look and taste just like the ones made in oil fryers. The air fryer serves up many ways to be useful in your life.

Consider:

- Do you find yourself short on time to cook?
- Are you having a hard time letting go of those fatty foods, but still want to lose weight?
- Are you always seeking to get a bang for your buck?

If you answered yes to any of these questions, then an air fryer may be for you.

Why You Should Use An Air Fryer

An air fryer can pretty much do it all. And by all, we mean fry, grill, bake, and roast. Equipped with sturdy plastic and metal material, the air fryer has many great benefits to offer.

Air Fryers Can:

- Cook multiple dishes at once
- Cut back on fatty oils
- Prepare a meal within minutes
- While every appliance has its cons, the air fryer doesn't offer many.
- The fryer may be bulky in weight, but its dimensions are slimmer than most fryers. An air fryer can barely take up any counter space.
- If you need fast, healthy, convenient, and tasty, then once again, an air fryer may be for you.

Air Fryer- Healthier

The biggest quality the air fryer offers is healthier dishes

In comparison to other fryers, air fryers were designed to specifically function without fattening oils and to produce food with up to 80 percent less fat than food cooked with other fryers. The air fryer can help you lose the weight, you've been dying to get rid of. While it can be difficult to let go of your favorite fried foods, an air fryer will let you have your cake and eat it too. You can still have your fried dishes, but at the same time, still conserve those calories and saturated fat. The air fryer can also grill, bake, and roast foods as well. Offering you an all in one combination, the air fryer is the perfect appliance for anyone looking to switch to a healthier lifestyle.

Fast And Quick

- If you're on a tight schedule, you may want to use an air fryer.
- Within minutes you can have crunchy golden fries or crispy chicken tenders.
- This fryer is perfect for people who are constantly on the go and do not have much time to prepare meals.
- With most air fryers, french fries can be prepared within 12 minutes.
- That cuts the time you spend in the kitchen by a tremendous amount.

Features

1. Temperature And Timer

- Avoid the waiting time for your fryer to decide when it wants to heat up.
- With an air fryer, once you power it on, the fryer will instantly heat.
- When using the appliance cold, that is, right after it has been off for a while (since last use) all you have to do is add three minutes to your cooking time to allow for it to heat up properly.
- The appliance is equipped with adjustable temperature control that allows you to set the temperature that can be altered for each of your

meals.

- Most fryers can go up to 200-300 degrees.
- Because the fryer can cook food at record times, it comes with a timer that can be pre-set with no more than 30 minutes.
- You can even check on the progress of your foods without messing up the set time. Simply pull out the pan, and the fryer will cause heating. When you replace the pan, heating will resume.
- When your meal is prepared and your timer runs out, the fryer will alert you with its ready sound indicator. But just in-case you can't make it to the fryer when the timer goes, the fryer will automatically switch off to help prevent your ingredients from overcooking and burning.

2. Food Separator

Some air fryers are supplied with a food separator that enables you to prepare multiple meals at once. For example, if you wanted to prepare frozen chicken nuggets and french fries, you could use the separator to cook both ingredients at the same time, all the while avoiding the worry of the flavors mixing. An air fryer is perfect for quick and easy, lunch and dinner combinations. It is recommended to pair similar ingredients together when using the separator. This will allow both foods to share a similar temperature setting.

3. Air Filter

Some air fryers are built with an integrated air filter that eliminates those unwanted vapors and food odors from spreading around your house. No more smelling like your favorite fried foods, the air filter will diffuse that hot oil steam that floats and sticks. You can now enjoy your fresh kitchen smell before, during, and after using your air fryer.

4. Cleaning

- No need to fret after using an air fryer, it was designed for hassle-free cleaning.
- The parts of the fryer are constructed of non-stick material.
- This prevents any food from sticking to surfaces that ultimately make

it hard to clean.
- It is recommended to soak the parts of the appliances before cleaning.
- All parts such as the grill, pan, and basket are removable and dishwasher friendly.
- After your ingredients are cooked to perfection, you can simply place your parts in the dishwasher for a quick and easy clean.

Tips on Cleaning an Air Fryer:

- Use detergent that specializes in dissolving oil.
- For a maximum and quick cleaning, leave the pan to soak in water and detergent for a few minutes.
- Avoid using metal utensils when cleaning the appliance to prevent scuffs and scratches on the material.
- Always let the fryer cool off for about 30 minutes before you wash it.

5. Cost-effective

Are there any cost-effective air fryers? For all that they can do, air fryers can be worth the cost. It has been highly questionable if the benefits of an air fryer are worth the expense. When you weigh your pros and cons, the air fryer surely leads with its pros. There aren't many fryers on the market that can fry, bake, grill and roast; and also promise you healthier meals. An air fryer saves you time, and could potentially save you money. Whether the air fryer is cost-effective for your life, is ultimately up to you.

The air fryer is a highly recommendable appliance to anyone starting a new diet, parents with busy schedules, or individuals who are always on the go. Deciding whether the investment is worth it, is all up to the purchaser. By weighing the air fryer advantages and the unique differences the air fryer has, compared to other fryers, you should be able to decide whether the air fryer has a lot to bring to the table.

Breakfast Recipes

1. Ham and Cheese Mini Quiche

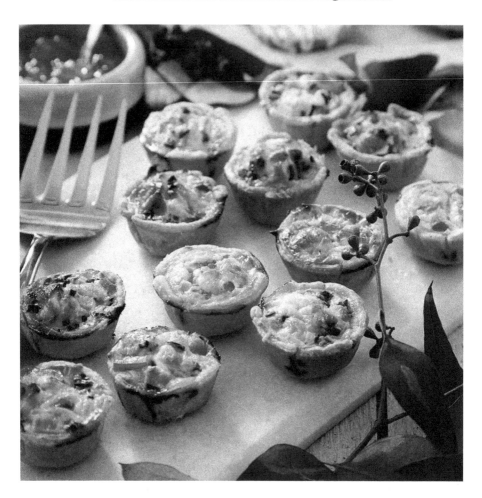

Prep Time: 30 minutes

Ingredients

- 1 shortcrust pastry
- 3 oz. chopped ham
- ½cup grated cheese

- 4 eggs, beaten
- 3 tbsp. greek yogurt
- ¼ tsp. garlic powder
- ¼ tsp. salt
- ¼ tsp. black pepper

Instructions

Preheat the air fryer to 330 degrees F.Take 8 ramekins and sprinkle them with flour to avoid sticking.cut the shortcrust pastry into 8 equal pieces to make 8 mini quiches.line your ramekins with the pastry.Combine all of the other **Ingredients** in a bowl.Divide the filling between the ramekins.Cook for 20 minutes

Nutrition Facts

Calories 365.7, Carbohydrates 21.4 g, Fat 20.4 g, Protein 8.9 g

2. Breakfast Banana Bread

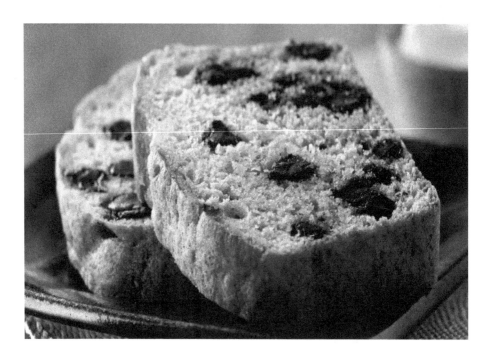

Prep Time: 50 minutes

Ingredients

- 1 cup plus
- 1 tbsp. flour
- ¼ tsp. baking soda
- 1 tsp. baking powder
- 1/3 cup sugar
- 2 mashed bananas
- ¼ cup vegetable oil
- 1 egg, beaten
- 1 tsp. vanilla extract
- ¾ cup chopped walnuts
- ¼ tsp. salt
- 2 tbsp. peanut butter2 tbsp. sour cream

Instructions

Preheat the air fryer to 330 degrees F.Spray a small baking dish with cooking spray or grease with butter.Combine the flour, salt, baking powder, and baking soda in a bowl.In another bowl combine bananas, oil, egg, peanut butter, vanilla, sugar, and sour cream. Combine both mixtures gently.Stir in the chopped walnuts.Pour the batter into the dish.Bake for 40 minutes.Let cool before serving.

Nutrition Facts

Calories 438, Carbohydrates 58 g, Fat 21 g, Protein 7.6

3. Baked Kale Omelet

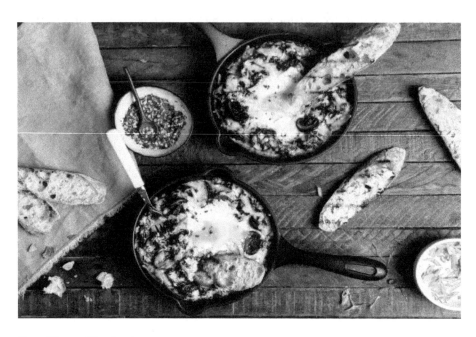

Prep Time: 15 minutes

Ingredients

- 3 eggs
- 3 tbsp. cottage cheese
- 3 tbsp. chopped kale
- ½ tbsp. chopped basil
- ½ tbsp. chopped parsleySalt and pepper, to taste
- 1 tsp. olive oil

Instructions

- Add oil to your air fryer and preheat it to 330 degrees F.
- Beat the eggs with some salt and pepper, in a bowl.
- Stir in the rest of the **Ingredients**.Pour the mixture into the air fryer and bake for 10 minutes

Nutrition Facts

Calories 294, Carbohydrates 3.9 g, Fat 19.5 g, Protein 24.7 g

4. Tasty Baked Eggs

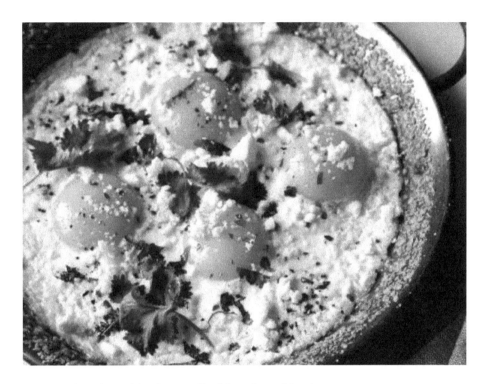

Preparation time: 10 minutes Cooking time: 20 minutes

Ingredients:

- 4 eggs
- 1 pound baby spinach, torn
- 7 ounces ham, chopped
- 4 tablespoons milk
- 1 tablespoon olive oil
- Cooking spray
- Salt and black pepper to the taste

Instructions:

- Heat up a pan with the oil over medium heat, add baby spinach, stir cook for a couple of minutes and take off heat.
- grease 4 ramekins with cooking spray and divide baby spinach and ham in each.

19

- Crack an egg in each ramekin, also divide milk, season with salt and pepper, place ramekins in preheated air fryer at 350 degrees F and bake for 20 minutes.
- Serve baked eggs for breakfast.

Nutrition Facts:

calories 321, fat 6, fiber 8, carbs 15, protein 12

5. Breakfast Egg Bowls

Preparation time: 10 minutes Cooking time: 20 minutes

Ingredients:

- 4 dinner rolls, tops cut off and insides scooped out
- 4 tablespoons heavy cream
- 4 eggs
- 4 tablespoons mixed chives and parsley
- Salt and black pepper to the taste
- 4 tablespoons parmesan, grated

Instructions:

- Arrange dinner rolls on a baking sheet and crack an egg in each.
- Divide heavy cream, mixed herbs in each roll and season with salt and pepper.
- Sprinkle parmesan on top of your rolls, place them in your air fryer and cook at 350 degrees F for 20 minutes.
- Divide your bread bowls on plates and serve for breakfast.

Nutrition Facts:

calories 238, fat 4, fiber 7, carbs 14, protein 7

Main & Lunch Recipes

6. Lunch Egg Rolls

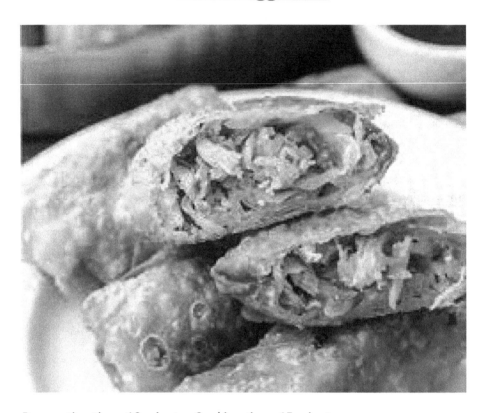

Preparation time: 10 minutes Cooking time: 15 minutes

Ingredients:

- ½ cup mushrooms, chopped
- ½ cup carrots, grated
- ½ cup zucchini, grated
- 2 green onions, chopped
- 2 tablespoons soy sauce
- 8 egg roll wrappers
- 1 eggs, whisked
- 1 tablespoon cornstarch

Instructions:

- In a bowl, mix carrots with mushrooms, zucchini, green onions and soy sauce and stir well.
- Arrange egg roll wrappers on a working surface, divide veggie mix on each and roll well.
- In a bowl, mix cornstarch with egg, whisk well and brush eggs rolls with this mix.
- Seal edges, place all rolls in your preheated air fryer and cook them at 370 degrees F for 15 minutes.
- Arrange them on a platter and serve them for lunch.

Nutrition Facts:

calories 172, fat 6, fiber 6, carbs 8, protein 7

7. <u>Veggie Toast</u>

Preparation time: 10 minutes Cooking time: 15 minutes

Ingredients:

- 1 red bell pepper, cut into thin strips
- 1 cup cremimi mushrooms, sliced
- 1 yellow squash, chopped
- 2 green onions, sliced
- 1 tablespoon olive oil
- 4 bread slices
- 2 tablespoons butter, soft
- ½ cup goat cheese, crumbled

Instructions:

- In a bowl, mix red bell pepper with mushrooms, squash, green onions and oil, toss, transfer to your air fryer, cook them at 350 degrees F for 10 minutes, shaking the fryer once and transfer them to a bowl.
- Spread butter on bread slices, place them in air fryer and cook them at 350 degrees F for 5 minutes.
- Divide veggie mix on each bread slice, top with crumbled cheese and serve for lunch.

Nutrition Facts:

calories 152, fat 3, fiber 4, carbs 7, protein 2

8. Stuffed Mushrooms

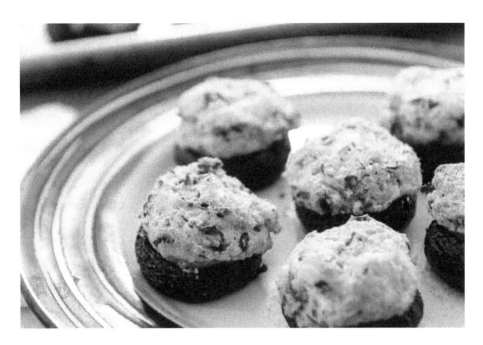

Preparation time: 10 minutes Cooking time: 20 minutes

Ingredients:

- 4 big Portobello mushroom caps
- 1 tablespoon olive oil
- ¼ cup ricotta cheese
- 5 tablespoons parmesan, grated
- 1 cup spinach, torn
- 1/3 cup bread crumbs
- ¼ teaspoon rosemary, chopped

Instructions:

- Rub mushrooms caps with the oil, place them in your air fryer's basket and cook them at 350 degrees F for 2 minutes.
- Meanwhile, in a bowl, mix half of the parmesan with ricotta, spinach, rosemary and bread crumbs and stir well.

- Stuff mushrooms with this mix, sprinkle the rest of the parmesan on top, place them in your air fryer's basket again and cook at 350 degrees F for 10 minutes.
- Divide them on plates and serve with a side salad for lunch.

Nutrition Facts:

calories 152, fat 4, fiber 7, carbs 9, protein 5

9. Quick Lunch Pizzas

Preparation time: 10 minutes Cooking time: 7 minutes

Ingredients:

- 4 pitas
- 1 tablespoon olive oil
- ¾ cup pizza sauce
- 4 ounces jarred mushrooms, sliced
- ½ teaspoon basil, dried
- 2 green onions, chopped
- 2 cup mozzarella, grated
- 1 cup grape tomatoes, sliced

Instructions:

- Spread pizza sauce on each pita bread, sprinkle green onions and basil, divide mushrooms and top with cheese.
- Arrange pita pizzas in your air fryer and cook them at 400 degrees F for 7 minutes.
- Top each pizza with tomato slices, divide among plates and serve.

Nutrition Facts:

calories 200, fat 4, fiber 6, carbs 7, protein 3

10. Gnocchi

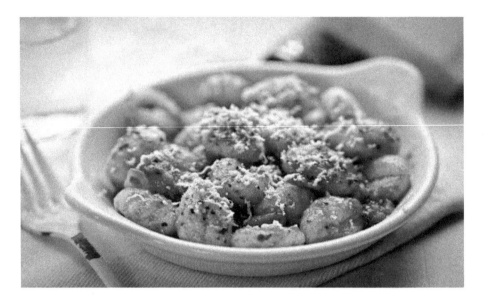

Preparation time: 10 minutes Cooking time: 17 minutes

Ingredients:

- 1 yellow onion, chopped
- 1 tablespoon olive oil
- 3 garlic cloves, minced
- 16 ounces gnocchi
- ¼ cup parmesan, grated
- 8 ounces spinach pesto

Instructions:

- grease your air fryer's pan with olive oil, add gnocchi, onion and garlic, toss, put pan in your air fryer and cook at 400 degrees F for 10 minutes.
- Add pesto, toss and cook for 7 minutes more at 350 degrees F.
- Divide among plates and serve for lunch.

Nutrition Facts: calories 200, fat 4, fiber 4, carbs 12, protein 4

11. Tuna and Zucchini Tortillas

Preparation time: 10 minutes Cooking time: 10 minutes

Ingredients:

4 corn tortillas

4 tablespoons butter, soft

6 ounces canned tuna, drained

1 cup zucchini, shredded

1/3 cup mayonnaise

2 tablespoons mustard

1 cup cheddar cheese, grated

Instructions:

- Spread butter on tortillas, place them in your air fryer's basket and cook them at 400 degrees F for 3 minutes.
- Meanwhile, in a bowl, mix tuna with zucchini, mayo and mustard and stir.
- Divide this mix on each tortilla, top with cheese, roll tortillas, place them in your air fryer's basket again and cook them at 400 degrees F for 4 minutes more.

Nutrition Facts:

calories 162, fat 4, fiber 8, carbs 9, protein 4

Side Dishes & Dinner Recipes

12. Fried Shrimp Sandwich Recipe

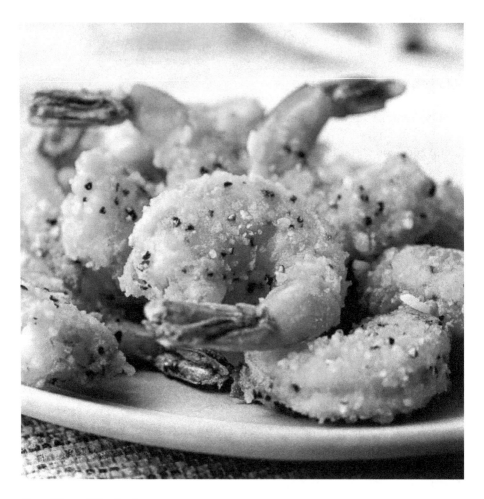

Prep Time: 20 minutes

Cook Time: 10 minutes

Total Time: 30 minutes

Ingredients

- 1 pound shrimp, deveined
- 1 teaspoon creole seasoning i used tony chachere
- 1/4 cup buttermilk
- 1/2 cup louisiana fish fry coating
- Cooking oil spray (if air frying) i use olive oil
- Canola or vegetable oil (if pan-frying) you will need enough oil to fill 2 inches of height in your frying pan.
- 4 french bread hoagie rolls i used 2 loaves, cut each in half
- 2 cups shredded iceberg lettuce
- 8 tomato slices

Remoulade Sauce

- 1/2 cup mayo I used reduced-fat
- 1 tsp minced garlic
- 1/2 lemon juice of
- 1 tsp Worcestershire
- 1/2 tsp Creole Seasoning I used Tony Chachere
- 1 tsp Dijon mustard
- 1 tsp hot sauce
- 1 green onion chopped

Instructions

Remoulade Sauce

- Combine all of the ingredients in a small bowl. Refrigerate before serving while the shrimp cooks.

Shrimp And Breading

- Marinate the shrimp in the Creole seasoning and buttermilk for 30 minutes. I like to use a sealable plastic bag to do this.
- Add the fish fry to a bowl. Remove the shrimp from the bags and dip each into the fish fry. Add the shrimp to the air fryer basket.

Pan Fry

- Heat a frying pan with 2 inches of oil to 350 degrees. Use a thermometer to test the heat.

- Fry the shrimp on both sides for 3-4 minutes until crisp.
- Remove the shrimp from the pan and drain the excess grease using paper towels.

Air Fryer

- Spray the air fryer basket with cooking oil. Add the shrimp to the air fryer basket.
- Spritz the shrimp with cooking oil.
- Cook the shrimp for 5 minutes at 400 degrees. Open the basket and flip the shrimp to the other side. Cook for an additional 3-5 minutes or until crisp.
- Assemble the Po Boy
- Spread the remoulade sauce on the French bread.
- Add the sliced tomato and lettuce, and then the shrimp.

Nutritional Facts

- Serving: 1serving | Calories: 437kcal | Carbohydrates: 55g | Protein: 24g | Fat: 12g

13. Easy Air Fryer Roasted Whole Chicken

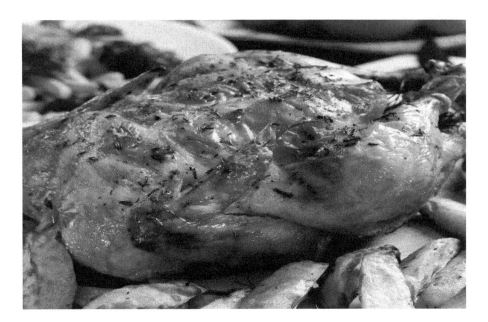

Prep Time: 15 minutes

Cook Time: 55 minutes

Resting: 15 minutes

Total Time: 1 hour 25 minutes

Ingredients

- 1 4.5-5 pounds whole chicken
- 1/2 fresh lemon
- 1/4 whole onion
- 4 sprigs of fresh thyme
- 4 sprigs of fresh rosemary
- Olive oil spray
- 1 teaspoon ground thyme i like to use ground thyme in addition to fresh thyme for optimal flavor.
- 1 teaspoon onion powder
- 1 teaspoon garlic powder

33

- Kosher salt to taste be sure to use kosher salt.

Instructions

- I purchased my whole chicken ready with the contents of the cavity removed. If your chicken still has the giblets inside of it, you will need to remove them before cooking.
- Stuff 1/2 of fresh-cut lemon and 1/4 of a chopped onion inside the cavity of the chicken along with the fresh rosemary and thyme.
- Make sure the chicken is completely dry on the outside. Pat dry with paper towels if necessary. A dry chicken will help it crisp in the air fryer with the olive oil.
- Spray olive oil onto both sides of the chicken using an oil sprayer.
- Sprinkle the seasonings throughout and onto both sides of the chicken. You may elect to only season the bottom side of the chicken at this step. Because you will need to flip the chicken during the air frying process, you will likely lose some of the seasonings at this stage. My preference is to season both sides initially, and then re-assess if more seasoning (usually salt is needed later).
- Line the air fryer with parchment paper. This makes for easy cleanup. Load the chicken into the air fryer basket with the breast side down.
- Air fry the chicken for 30 minutes at 330 degrees.
- Open the air fryer and flip the chicken. I gripped the chicken cavity with tongs to flip.
- Re-assess if more seasoning is needed on the breasts, legs, and wings. Add additional if necessary.
- Air fry for an additional 20-25 minutes until the chicken reaches an internal temperature of 165 degrees. Use a meat thermometer.
- This step is important. Place the meat thermometer in the thickest part of the chicken, which is typically the chicken thigh area. I like to test the breast too, just to ensure the entire chicken is fully cooked.
- Remove the chicken from the air fryer basket and place it on a plate to rest for at least 15 minutes before cutting into the chicken. This will allow the moisture to redistribute throughout the chicken before you cut into it.

Nutrition Facts

- Calories: 340kcal | Carbohydrates: 2g | Protein: 33g | Fat: 22g

14.   Air Fryer Beef Taco Fried Egg Rolls

Prep Time: 15 minutes

Cook Time: 25 minutes

Total Time: 40 minutes

Servings: 8

Ingredients

- 1 pound ground beef
- 16 egg roll wrappers i used wing hing brand
- 1/2 cup chopped onion i used red onion.
- 2 garlic cloves minced
- 16 oz can diced tomatoes and chilies i used mexican rotel.
- 8 oz refried black beans i used fat-free and 1/2 of a 16oz can.
- 1 cup shredded mexican cheese
- 1/2 cup whole kernel corn i used frozen
- Cooking oil spray
- Homemade taco seasoning
- 1 tablespoon chili powder
- 1 teaspoon cumin
- 1 teaspoon smoked paprika
- Salt and pepper to taste

Instructions

- Add the ground beef to a skillet on medium-high heat along with the salt, pepper, and taco seasoning. Cook until browned while breaking the beef into smaller chunks.
- Once the meat has started to brown add the chopped onions and garlic. Cook until the onions become fragrant.
- Add the diced tomatoes and chilis, Mexican cheese, beans, and corn. Stir to ensure the mixture is combined.
- Lay the egg roll wrappers on a flat surface. Dip a cooking brush in water. Glaze each of the egg roll wrappers with the wet brush along the edges. This will soften the crust and make it easier to roll.

- Load 2 tablespoons of the mixture into each of the wrappers. Do not overstuff. Depending on the brand of egg roll wrappers you use, you may need to double wrap the egg rolls.
- Fold the wrappers diagonally to close. Press firmly on the area with the filling, cup it to secure it in place. Fold in the left and right sides as triangles. Fold the final layer over the top to close. Use the cooking brush to wet the area and secure it in place.
- Spray the air fryer basket with cooking oil.
- Load the egg rolls into the basket of the Air Fryer. Spray each egg roll with cooking oil.
- Cook for 8 minutes at 400 degrees. Flip the egg rolls. Cook for an additional 4 minutes or until browned and crisp.

Nutrition Facts

- Calories: 348kcal | Carbohydrates: 38g | Protein: 24g | Fat: 11g

15. Air Fryer Beef Taco Fried Egg Rolls

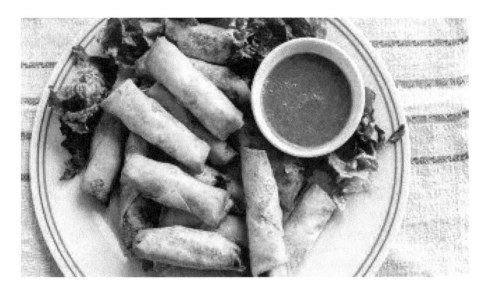

Prep Time: 15 minutes

Cook Time: 25 minutes

Total Time: 40 minutes

Servings: 8

Ingredients

- 1 pound ground beef
- 16 egg roll wrappers i used wing hing brand
- 1/2 cup chopped onion i used red onion.
- 2 garlic cloves minced
- 16 oz can diced tomatoes and chilies i used mexican rotel.
- 8 oz refried black beans i used fat-free and 1/2 of a 16oz can.
- 1 cup shredded mexican cheese
- 1/2 cup whole kernel corn i used frozen
- Cooking oil spray

Homemade Taco Seasoning

- 1 tablespoon chili powder
- 1 teaspoon cumin
- 1 teaspoon smoked paprika
- Salt and pepper to taste

Instructions

- Add the ground beef to a skillet on medium-high heat along with the salt, pepper, and taco seasoning. Cook until browned while breaking the beef into smaller chunks.
- Once the meat has started to brown add the chopped onions and garlic. Cook until the onions become fragrant.
- Add the diced tomatoes and chilis, Mexican cheese, beans, and corn. Stir to ensure the mixture is combined.
- Lay the egg roll wrappers on a flat surface. Dip a cooking brush in water. Glaze each of the egg roll wrappers with the wet brush along the edges. This will soften the crust and make it easier to roll.
- Load 2 tablespoons of the mixture into each of the wrappers. Do not overstuff. Depending on the brand of egg roll wrappers you use, you may need to double wrap the egg rolls.
- Fold the wrappers diagonally to close. Press firmly on the area with the filling, cup it to secure it in place. Fold in the left and right sides as triangles. Fold the final layer over the top to close. Use the cooking brush to wet the area and secure it in place.
- Spray the air fryer basket with cooking oil.
- Load the egg rolls into the basket of the Air Fryer. Spray each egg roll with cooking oil.
- Cook for 8 minutes at 400 degrees. Flip the egg rolls. Cook for an additional 4 minutes or until browned and crisp.

Nutrition Facts

- Calories: 348kcal | Carbohydrates: 38g | Protein: 24g | Fat: 11g

16.   Easy Crispy Garlic Parmesan Chicken Wings

Prep Time: 15 minutes

Cook Time: 45 minutes

Total Time:1 hour

Servings: 4

Ingredients

- 1 pound chicken wings (drummettes)
- 1/2 cup flour see recipe notes for low carb substitute.
- 1/2 cup grated parmesan divided into two 1/4 cup servings
- 1/2 tablespoon mccormicks grill mates chicken seasoning you can use your favorite chicken rub.
- Salt and pepper to taste
- Cooking oil i use olive oil.
- 3 garlic cloves minced
- 1 tablespoon butter
- 1 tablespoon olive oil

Instructions

- Oven and Baking Instructions
- Preheat the oven to 375 degrees.
- Pat the chicken dry and place it on a large bowl or plastic bag.
- Add the flour, 1/4 cup of grated parmesan, chicken seasoning, salt, and pepper to the chicken. Ensure the chicken is fully coated.
- Line a sheet pan with parchment paper and add the wings. Spritz the chicken wings with cooking oil.
- Bake the wings for 20 minutes and then open and flip the wings. Spritz with cooking oil. Bake for an additional 10 minutes.
- Heat a saucepan on medium-high heat. Add the butter, 1 tablespoon of olive oil, garlic, and 1/4 cup of grated parmesan.
- Cook for 2-3 minutes until the butter and cheese have melted.

- Remove the chicken from the oven and drizzle the wings in the garlic parmesan sauce.
- Return the chicken to the oven. Bake for an additional 10-15 minutes.
- Garnish with parsley and parmesan if you wish.

Air Fryer Instructions

- Pat the chicken dry and place it on a large bowl or plastic bag.
- Add the flour, 1/4 cup of grated parmesan, chicken seasoning, salt, and pepper to the chicken. Ensure the chicken is fully coated.
- Line the air fryer basket with air fryer parchment paper. Place the chicken on the parchment paper. Spritz the chicken with olive oil.
- Air fry for 15 minutes at 400 degrees.
- Open the air fryer and flip the chicken. Spritz the chicken with cooking oil. Cook for an additional 5 minutes.
- Heat a saucepan on medium-high heat. Add the butter, 1 tablespoon of olive oil, garlic, and 1/4 cup of grated parmesan.
- Cook for 2-3 minutes until the butter and cheese have melted.
- Remove the chicken from the air fryer and drizzle it with the garlic parmesan butter.
- Return the chicken to the air fryer. Air fryer for an additional 3-4 minutes on 400 degrees.
- Garnish with parsley and parmesan if you wish.

Nutrition Facts

- Calories: 374kcal | Carbohydrates: 11g | Protein: 26g | Fat: 24g

17.   Air Fryer Crispy Crab Rangoon

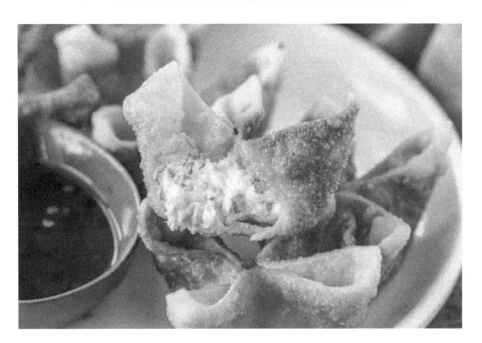

Prep Time: 15 minutes

Cook Time: 15 minutes

Total Time: 30 minutes

Ingredients

- 4 or 6 oz cream cheese, softened If you prefer creamy crab rangoon use 6 oz
- 4 or 6 oz lump crab meat If you prefer your crab rangoon to have more cream cheese and less crab, use 4 oz. Seafood lovers may want to go for 6 oz
- 2 green onions, chopped
- 21 wonton wrappers
- 2 garlic cloves, minced
- 1 teaspoon Worcestershire sauce
- Salt and pepper to taste
- Cooking oil I use olive oil.

41

Instructions

- You can soften your cream cheese by heating it in the microwave for 20 seconds.
- Combine the cream cheese, green onions, crab meat, Worcestershire sauce, salt, pepper, and garlic in a small bowl. Stir to mix well.
- Layout the wonton wrappers on a working surface. I used a large, bamboo cutting board. Moisten each of the wrappers with water. I use a cooking brush, and brush it along all of the edges.
- Load about a teaspoon and a half of filling onto each wrapper. Be careful not to overfill.
- Fold each wrapper diagonally across to form a triangle. From there bring up the two opposite corners toward each other. Don't close the wrapper yet. Bring up the other two opposite sides, pushing out any air. Squeeze each of the edges together. Be sure to check out the recipe video above for illustration.
- Spritz the air fryer basket with cooking oil.
- Load the crab rangoon into the air fryer basket. Do not stack or overfill. Cook in batches if needed.
- Spritz with oil.
- Place the Air Fryer at 370 degrees. Cook for 10 minutes.
- Open and flip the crab rangoon. Cook for an additional 2-5 minutes until they have reached your desired level of golden brown and crisp.
- Remove the crab rangoon from the air fryer and serve with your desired dipping sauce.

Nutrition Facts

- Calories: 98kcal | Carbohydrates: 12g | Protein: 7g | Fat: 3g

Seafoods Recipes

18. Frozen sesame Fish Fillets

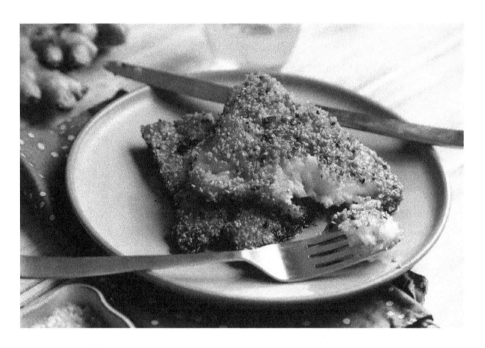

Prep Time: 20 minutes

Ingredients:

5 frozen fish fillets

5 biscuits, crumbled

3 tbsp. flour

1 egg, beaten

Pinch of salt and Pinch of black pepper

¼ tsp. rosemary

3 tbsp. olive oil divided

A handful of sesame seeds

Instructions:

Preheat the air fryer to 390 degrees F. Combine the flour, pepper and salt, in a shallow bowl.In another shallow bowl, combine the sesame seeds, crumbled biscuits, oil, and rosemary. Dip the fish fillets into the flour mixture first, then into the beaten egg, and finally, coat them with the sesame mixture.Arrange them inside the air fryer on a sheet of aluminum foil.Cook the fish for 8 minutes.Flip the fillets over and cook for additional 4 minutes.

Nutrition Facts

Calories 257.6, Carbohydrates 16.4 g, Fat 14 g, Protein 19.1 g

19. **Fish Tacos**

Prep Time: 15 minutes

Ingredients:

4 corn tortillas

1 halibut fillet

2 tbsp. olive oil1

½ cup flour, divided

1 can of beer

1 tsp. salt

4 tbsp. peach salsa

4 tsp. chopped cilantro1 tsp. baking powder

Instructions:

Preheat the air fryer to 390 degrees F. Combine 1 cup of flour, baking, powder and salt. Pour in some of the beer, enough to form a batter-like consistency. Save the rest of the beer to gulp with the taco. Slice the fillet into 4 strips and toss them in half cup of flour. Dip them into the beer batter and arrange on a lined baking sheet. Place in the air fryer and cook for 8 minutes. Meanwhile, spread the peach salsa on the tortillas.Top each tortilla with one fish strip and 1 tsp. chopped cilantro.

Nutrition Facts

Calories 369, Carbohydrates 52 g, Fat 8.8 g, Protein 14.2 g

20. Peppery and Lemony Haddock

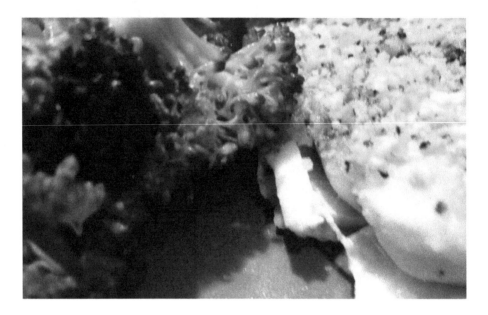

Prep Time: 15 minutes

Ingredients:

4 haddock fillets

1 cup breadcrumbs

2 tbsp. lemon juice

½ tsp. black pepper

¼ cup dry instant potato flakes1 egg, beaten¼ cup Parmesan cheese

3 tbsp. flour

¼ tsp. salt

Instructions:

Combine the flour, pepper and salt, in a small shallow bowl. In another bowl, combine the lemon, breadcrumbs, Parmesan, and potato flakes. Dip the fillets in the flour first, then in the beaten egg, and coat them with the lemony crumbs. Arrange on a lined sheet and place in the air fryer. Air fry for about 8 to 10 minutes at 370 degrees F.

Nutrition Facts

Calories 310.6, Carbohydrates 26.9 g, Fat 6.3 g, Protein 34.8 g

21. Soy Sauce Glazed Cod

Prep Time: 15 minutes

Ingredients:

1 cod fillet1 tsp. olive oil

Pinch of sea salt

Pinch of pepper

1 tbsp. soy sauce

Dash of sesame oil

¼ tsp. ginger powder

¼ tsp. honey

Instructions:

Preheat the air fryer to 370 degrees F. Combine the olive oil, salt and pepper, and brush that mixture over the cod. Place the cod onto an aluminum sheet and into the air fryer.Cook for about 6 minutes.Meanwhile, combine the soy sauce, ginger, honey, and sesame oil.Brush the glaze over the cod.Flip the fillet over and cook for additional 3 minutes.

Nutrition Facts

Calories 148, Carbohydrates 2.9 g, Fat 5.8 g, Protein 21 g

22. Salmon Cakes

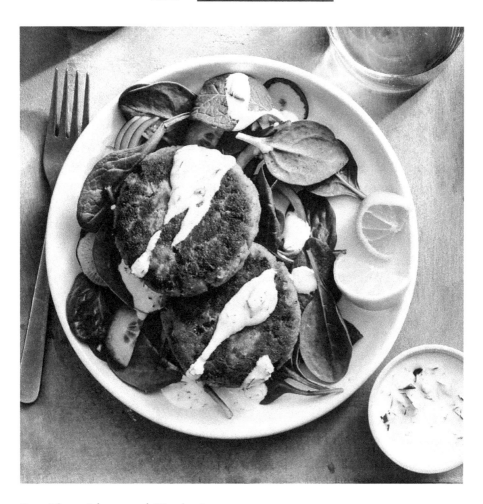

Prep Time: 1 hour and 15 minutes

Ingredients:

10 oz. cooked salmon

14 oz. boiled and mashed potatoes

2 oz. flour

Handful capers

Handful chopped parsley

1 tsp. olive oil

Zest of 1 lemon

Instructions:

Place the mashed potatoes in a large bowl and flake the salmon over.Stir in capers, parsley, and lemon zest.Shape small cakes out of the mixture.Dust them with flour and place in the fridge to set, for about 1 hour.Preheat the air fryer to 350 degrees F.Brush the olive oil over the basket's bottom and add the cakes.Cook for about 7 minutes.

Nutrition Facts

Calories 240.8, Carbohydrates 28.6 g, Fat 6.4 g, Protein 17.7 g

23. Rosemary Garlicky Prawns

Prep Time:

1 h 15 minutes

Ingredients:

8 large prawns

3 garlic cloves, minced

1 rosemary sprig, chopped

½ tbsp. melted butter

Salt and pepper, to taste

Instructions:

Combine the garlic, butter, rosemary, and some salt and pepper, in a bowl.Add the prawns to the bowl and mix to coat them well.Cover the bowl and refrigerate for about an hour.Preheat the air fryer to 350 degrees F.Cook for about 6 minutes.Increase the temperature to 390 degrees, and cook for one more minute.

Nutrition Facts

Calories 152.2, Carbohydrates 1.5 g, Fat 2.9 g, Protein 0.3 g

24. Parmesan Tilapia

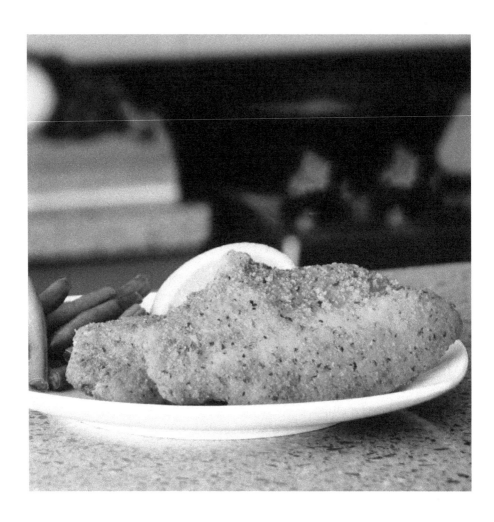

Prep Time: 15 minutes

Ingredients:

¾ cup grated Parmesan cheese

1 tbsp. olive oil

2 tsp. paprika

1 tbsp. chopped parsley

¼ tsp. garlic powder¼ tsp. salt4 tilapia fillets

Instructions:

Preheat the air fryer to 350 degrees F.Mix parsley, Parmesan, garlic, salt, and paprika in a shallow bowl.Brush the olive oil over the fillets, and then coat them with the Parmesan mixture.Place the tilapia onto a lined baking sheet, and then into the air fryer.Cook for about 4 to 5 minutes on all sides.

Nutrition Facts

Calories 228.4, Carbohydrates 1.3 g, Fat 11.1 g, Protein 31.9 g

25. Cheesy Bacon Wrapped Shrimp

Preparation time: 20mins

Ingredients

- 16 extra-large raw shrimp, peeled, deveined, and butterflied
- 16 (1 in) cubes cheddar jack cheese
- 16 slices of bacon, cooked half way
- ¼ cup BBQ sauce

Instructions

- Preheat the air fryer to 350 degrees F.
- Stuff each shrimp with a cheese cube and wrap with a slice of bacon.
- Secure the bacon to the shrimp with a toothpick.
- Brush the wrapped shrimp with BBQ sauce and place in the air fryer.
- Cook for 6 minutes.
- Remove and brush with additional BBQ sauce.

Nutrition facts:

Calorie 110

Protein 11g

26. Salmon Quiche

Preparation time: 60mins

Ingredients

- 2 cups salmon, skinless and cubed
- 1 tsp. salt
- ¼ tsp. ground black pepper
- 1 (9 in) premade pie crust
- 3 large eggs
- 1 tbsp. Dijon mustard
- ¼ cup green onion, chopped
- ½ cup shredded mozzarella cheese
- 4 tbsp. heavy cream

Instructions

- Preheat the air fryer to a temperature of 350 degrees F
- Then, Season the salmon with salt and pepper to your taste. Set aside. Place the pre-made pie crust into individual quiche pans and press into the sides of the pans.
- Trim off any overhanging crust. Trim the dough onto the edges of the pan you intend to use or just let it stick out.
- Place the cubed salmon into the crust and top with the green onion and mozzarella. In a mixing bowl, combine the heavy cream, eggs, and mustard.
- Carefully pour over the salmon, being careful not cause the mixture to overflow.
- Carefully slide the quiche into the fryer basket and cook for 20 minutes.
- Let rest for 10 minutes before serving.

Nutrition facts:

Calorie 287.2,Fats 13g,Fiber 0.4g,Carbs 11.4g,Protein 29.5g

27.   Cedar Plank Salmon

Preparation time: 30mins

Ingredients

- 4 untreated cedar planks
- 1½ tbsp. of rice vinegar
- 2 tbsp. sesame oil
- ½ cup soy sauce
- ¼ cup green onions, chopped
- 3 cloves garlic, minced
- 1 tbsp. fresh ginger grated
- 2 lb. of salmon fillets, skin removed

Instructions

Submerge the cedar planks in water and soak for 2 hours.

- In a shallow dish, combine all **Ingredients** except salmon and mix well.
- Add the salmon to the marinade and coat each side.
- Marinate, refrigerated, for 30minutes.
- Preheat fryer to 350 degrees F.
- Remove the cedar planks from the water and pat dry.
- Place on the fryer basket and place the salmon on top
- Cook for 15 minutes. Serve and enjoy

Nutrition facts:

Calorie 540

Fats 32g

Fiber 3g

Carbs 28g

Protein 38g

28. Chinese Mushroom Tilapia

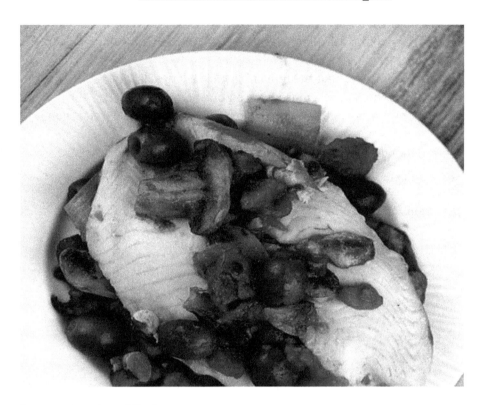

Preparation time: 20mins

Ingredients

- ½ cup yellow onion, sliced thin
- 2 cloves garlic, minced
- 4 (8oz) fillets tilapia
- 2½ tsps. of salt
- 2 tbsp. olive oil
- 2 cups sliced mushrooms
- 4 tbsp. soy sauce
- 1 tsp. red chili flakes
- 1 tbsp. honey 2 tbsp. rice vinegar

Instructions

- Preheat the fryer to 350 degrees F.
- Season the fish with half the salt and drizzle with half the oil. Cook for 15 minutes.
- Meanwhile, heat the remaining oil in a large skillet.
- Once hot add the mushroom onion and garlic.
- Cook until onions are soft. Stir in the soy sauce, chili flakes, honey, and vinegar. Simmer for 1 minute.
- Remove fish from the fryer and top with mushroom sauce.

Serve and enjoy!

Nutrition facts:

Calorie 57,Fats 3.5g,Fiber 1.8g,Carbs 1.7g,Protein 1.8g

29.   Air Fried Spinach Fish

Preparation time: 20mins

Ingredients

- 1 cup spinach leaves, wilted
- 2 cups flour
- 1 tsp. salt
- ½ tsp. ground black pepper
- 2 tbsp. olive oil
- 1 large egg
- 4 (6oz) filets perch
- 1 tbsp. lemon juice

Instructions

- Preheat the fryer to 370 degrees F.
- In a bowl, combine the spinach, flour, salt, pepper, and egg.
- Dip each filet in the batter and place on the fryer tray.
- Drizzle with olive oil. Cook for 12 minutes.
- Remove and drizzle with lemon juice.

Nutrition facts:

Calorie 227.8

Fats 5.1g

Fiber 1.8g

Carbs 14.2g

Protein 1.8g

30. Air Fryer Fried Louisiana Shrimp Po Boy with Remoulade Sauce

Preparation time: 30mins

Ingredients

- 4 French bread hoagie rolls I used 2 loaves, cut each in half
- 2 cups shredded lettuce
- 1 pound shrimp, deveined I usually go for the biggest shrimp I can find because they shrink a little when you cook them
- 1/2 cup Louisiana Fish Fry
- 1/4 cup buttermilk
- 8 tomato slices
- 1 tsps. Creole Seasoning I used Cony Chachere
- 1 tsps. butter optional

Remoulade Sauce

- 1/2 cup mayo I used reduced-fat
- 1 tsp. minced garlic
- 1/2 lemon juice of
- 1 tsp. Worcestershire
- 1/2 tsp. Creole Seasoning I used Cony Chachere
- 1 tsp. Dijon mustard
- 1 tsp. hot sauce
- 1 green onion chopped

Instructions

- Remoulade Sauce
- Combine all of the **Ingredients** in a small bowl. Refrigerate prior to serving while the shrimp cooks.
- Shrimp Po Boy
- Season the shrimp with the seasonings.
- Pour the buttermilk in a bowl. Dip each of the shrimp in the buttermilk. Place the shrimp in a Ziploc bag and in the fridge to marinate. Marinate for at least 30 minutes. I prefer overnight.

- Add the fish fry to a bowl. Remove the shrimp from the bags and dip each into the fish fry. Add the shrimp to Air Fryer basket.
- Preheat Air Fryer to 400 degrees.
- Spray the shrimp with olive oil. Do not spray directly on the shrimp. The fish fry will go flying. Keep a nice distance.
- Cook the shrimp for 5 minutes. Open the basket and flip the shrimp to the other side. Cook for an additional 5 minutes or until crisp.
- Preheat oven to 325 degrees. Place the sliced bread on a sheet pan.
- Allow the bread to toast for a couple of minutes.
- Optional step if you prefer butter: Melt the butter in the microwave. Using a cooking brush, spread the butter over the bottom of the French bread.
- Assemble the po boy. Spread the remoulade sauce on the French bread. Add the sliced tomato and lettuce, and then the shrimp.

Nutrition facts:

Calorie 437

Fats 12g

Fiber 1.8g

Carbs 32g

Protein 28g

31. Air Fryer Fried Catfish

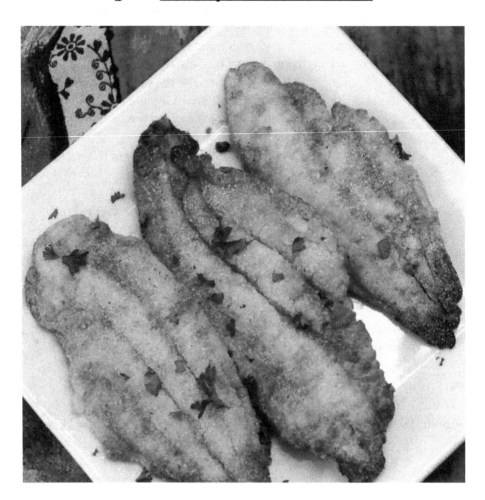

Preparation time: 65mins

Ingredients

- 4 catfish fillets
- 1/4 cup seasoned fish fry I used Louisiana
- 1 tbsp. olive oil
- 1 tbsp. chopped parsley optional

Instructions

- Preheat Air Fryer to 400 degrees.
- Rinse the catfish and pat dry.
- Pour the fish fry seasoning in a large Ziploc bag.
- Add the catfish to the bag, one at a time. Seal the bag and shake. Ensure the entire filet is coated with seasoning.
- Spray olive oil on the top of each filet.
- Place the filet in the Air Fryer basket. (Due to the size of my fillets, I cooked each one at a time). Close and cook for 10 minutes.
- Flip the fish. Cook for an additional 10 minutes.
- Flip the fish.
- Cook for an additional 2-3 minutes or until desired crispness.
- Top with parsley

Nutrition facts:

Calorie 208

Fats 11.2g

Fiber 0.5g

Carbs 15.4g

Protein 13.3g

Snacks And Appetizers

32.   Pita Pizza

Preparation Time: 5 minutes

Ingredients:

- ¼ cup pizza sauce
- 1 large thin pita bread
- ¼ cup sliced mushrooms
- 10 black olives
- ¼ cup green pepper
- ½ cup fat free mozzarella
- Pinch of pizza seasoning
- 2 teaspoon parmesan

Instructions:

Preheat oven to broil.

Spread the pita with pizza sauce.

Layer on the vegetables and the top with the cheese and seasoning.

Spray with cooking spray.

Broil for 2 minutes.

Nutritional Value

Calories 317

Fat 11g

Protein 15g

Carbohydrates 39g

33. Vegan Bacon Wrapped Mini Breakfast Burritos

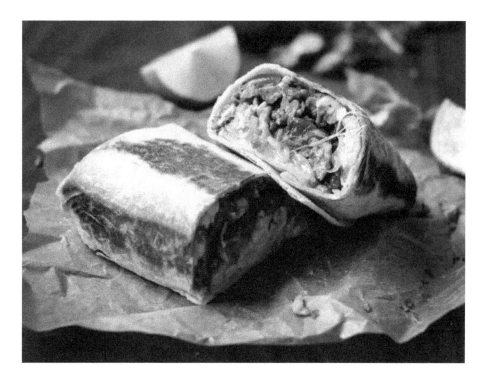

Preparation time: 20 mins

Ingredients

- 2 tablespoons cashew butter
- 6-8 stalks fresh asparagus
- handful spinach, kale, other greens
- 2 – 3 tablespoons tamari
- 2 servings Vegan Egg scramble or Tofu Scramble
- veggie add-ins:
- ⅓ cup roasted sweet potato cubes
- 1 – 2 tablespoons liquid smoke
- 1-2 tablespoons water
- 4 pieces of rice paper
- 8 strips roasted red pepper

- 1 small tree broccoli, sautéed

Instructions

Preheat Air Fryer to 350 °F. In a small shallow bowl, whisk together cashew butter, tamari, liquid smoke, and water. Set aside.

Prepare all fillings to assemble rolls.

Rice Paper Hydrating Technique: have a large plate/surface ready to fill/roll wrapper. Hold one rice paper under water faucet running cool water, getting both sides of wrapper wet, for just a few seconds. Remove from water and while still firm, place on a plate to fill – rice paper will soften as it sits, but will not be so soft that it sticks to the surface or rips when handling.

Fill by placing **Ingredients** just off from the middle, leaving sides of rice paper free. Fold two sides in like a burrito, roll from ingredient side to other side, and seal. Dip each roll into cashew - liquid smoke mixture, coating completely. Arrange rolls on parchment Air fryer.

Cook at 350 °F for 8-10 minutes, or until crisp.

Serve warm

Nutrition facts:

Calorie 394.9

Fats 25.1g

Fiber 11g

Carbs 19.5g

Protein 21g

34. Air fryer Baked Thai Peanut Chicken Egg Rolls

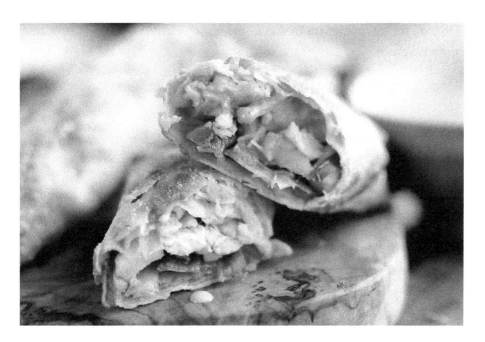

Preparation time: 18 mins

Ingredients

- 1 medium carrot, very thinly sliced or ribboned
- 3 green onions, chopped
- 4 egg roll wrappers
- 2 c. rotisserie chicken, shredded
- ¼ c. Thai peanut sauce
- ¼ red bell pepper, julienned
- non-stick cooking spray or sesame oil

Instructions

Preheat Air fryer to 390° or oven to 425°.

In a small bowl, toss the chicken with the Thai peanut sauce.

Lay the egg roll wrappers out on a clean dry surface. Over the bottom third of an egg roll wrapper, arrange ¼ the carrot, bell pepper, and onions. Spoon ½ cup of the chicken mixture over the vegetables.

Moisten the outside edges of the wrapper with water. Fold the sides of the wrapper toward the center and roll tightly.

Repeat with remaining wrappers. (Keep remaining wrappers covered with a damp paper towel until ready to use.)

Spray the assembled egg rolls with non-stick cooking spray. Turn them over and spray the backsides as well.

Place the egg rolls in the Air fryer and bake at 390° for 6-8 minutes or until they are crispy and golden brown.

(If you are baking the egg rolls in an oven, place the seam side down on a baking sheet coated with cooking spray. Bake at 425° for 45-20 minutes.)

Slice in half and serve with additional Thai Peanut Sauce for dipping.

Nutrition facts:

Calorie 235

Fats 7g

Fiber 1g

Carbs 17g

Protein 21g

35. Air Fryer Cheese Sticks Recipe

Preparation time: 22 mins

Ingredients

- 1/4 cup grated parmesan cheese
- 1 tsp. Italian Seasoning
- 1 tsp. garlic powder
- 6 snack-size cheese sticks (the individual ones you buy for kids)
- 2 large eggs
- 1/4 cup whole wheat flour (any type - pastry or white whole wheat work well)
- 1/4 tsp. ground rosemary

Instructions

Unwrap your cheese sticks and set aside.

Crack and beat your eggs with a fork a shallow bowl that is wide enough to fit the length of the cheese sticks.

In another bowl (or plate), mix the flour, cheese, and seasonings.

Roll the cheese sticks in the egg, then in the batter. Repeat until the cheese sticks are well coated.

Place them in the basket of your air fryer, ensuring they don't touch.

Cook to your air fryer's **Instructions**. On mine, the temperature was 370 F. for 6-7 minutes.

Serve with a clean marinara or ketchup (or ranch dressing!)

Nutrition facts:

Calorie 50 Fats 2g Fiber 0g Carbs 3g Protein 3g

36. Healthy Air Fried Chicken Meatballs

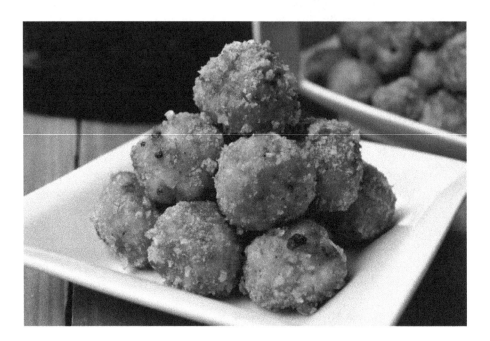

Prep Time: 20 mins

Total Time: 25 mins

Ingredients

- 1 Pound of ground chicken
- 2 Finely chopped green onions
- ½ Cup of chopped cilantro
- 1 Tbsp of Hoisin Sauce
- 1 Tbsp of soy sauce
- 1 tsp of Sriracha
- 1 tsp of sesame oil
- ¼ Cup of unsweetened shredded coconut
- 1 Pinch of salt
- 1 Pinch of ground black pepper

Instructions:

Heat your Air Fryer to a temperature of about 350°F.

Mix all your **Ingredients** in a large bowl. Line your Air Fryer baking pan with a paper sheet. With spoon, scoop the mixture into small rounds.

Place the baking pan in your Air Fryer; then lock the lid of your Air Fryer. Set the timer to about 10 to 12 minutes and the temperature to about 380° F

When the timer beeps; turn off your Air Fryer; then remove the pan from the air fryer and set it aside to cool for about 5 minutes.

Serve and enjoy your appetizing chicken balls!

Nutrition facts:

Calories 279 ,Total Fats 13 g ,Carbs: 9.8 g,Protein 28.8 g,Sugar 1.5 g

Fiber 0.5 g

37. Mexican Empanada

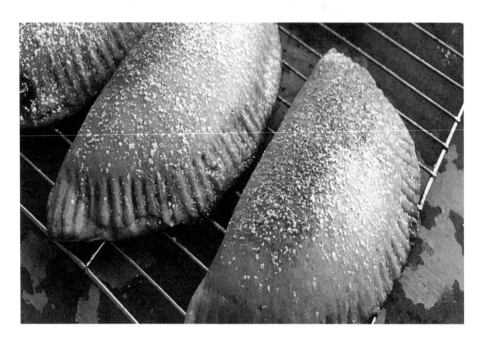

Preparation time: 40 mins

Ingredients

- 1 shallot, chopped
- 7 ounces store-bought pizza dough
- ¼ red bell pepper, diced
- 4 ½ ounces chorizo, cubed
- 2 tbsp. parsley

Instructions:

In a pan over medium heat, sauté the pepper, shallots, and chorizo together for 3-5 minutes.

Turn the heat off before adding in the parsley.

Take 20 small rounds from the dough. You may use a cookie cutter if you ant.

Scoop out some of the chorizo mixture and place it on the center of each round of dough. Fold and secure the edges. Do the same for the rest of the Ingredients. Cook the empanadas in the air fryer at 390°F for 10-12 minutes.

Nutrition facts:

Calorie 283,Fats 22g,Fiber 1g,Carbs 5g,Protein 17g

38. Mushroom-Salami Pizza

Preparation time: 30mins

Ingredients

- 1 tsp. butter, melted
- ¼ cup tomato sauce
- 1 small, store-bought
- 8-in pizza dough
- ½ ball of mozzarella sliced thinly
- ½ tbsp. olive oil
- 3 mushrooms, sliced
- 1 ½ ounces salami, cut into strips
- Pepper to taste
- 2 tsp. dried oregano
- 2 tbsp. Parmesan cheese, grated

Instructions:

Press and pat the dough on a well-greased pizza pan. Use the butter to grease the pan.

Spread the sauce all over the dough then top it all with cheese.

Now, sprinkle the mushrooms and salami over the pizza base.

Season it with oregano, pepper, and cheese.

Cook it in a preheated air-fryer at 390°F for 12 minutes.

Nutrition facts:

Calorie 233.9

Fats 9g

Fiber 1.3g

Carbs 26.3g

Meat Recipes

39. Air Fryer Steak

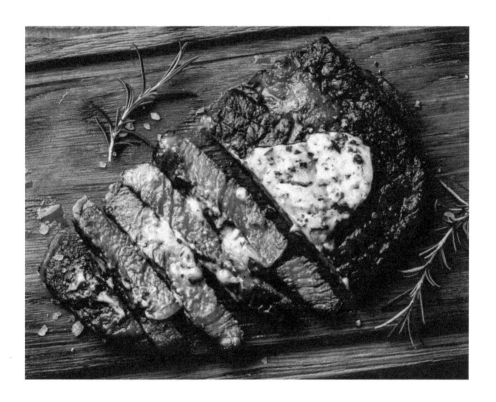

Prep Time: 5 mins ,Cook Time: 25 mins ,Total Time: 30 mins

Ingredients

- 2 (6 oz.) ((170g)) steaks, 3/4" thick rinsed and patted dry
- 1 teaspoon (5 ml) olive oil, to coat
- 1/2 teaspoon (0.5) garlic powder (optional)
- Salt, to taste
- Pepper, to taste
- Butter

Instructions

- Lightly coat steaks with olive oil. Season both sides of steaks with garlic powder (optional), salt, and pepper (we'll usually season liberally with salt & pepper).
- Preheat the Air Fryer at 400°F for 4 minutes.
- Air Fry for 400°F for 10-18 minutes, flipping halfway through (cooking time depends on how thick and cold the steaks are plus how do you prefer your steaks).
- If you want steaks to be cooked more, add additional 3-6 minutes of cooking time.
- Add a pat of butter on top of the steak, cover with foil, and allow the steak to rest for 5 minutes.
- Season with additional salt and pepper, if needed. Serve immediately.

Nutrition Facts

- Calories: 373kcal | Protein: 34g | Fat: 26g | Saturated Fat: 10g | Cholesterol: 103mg | Sodium: 88mg | Potassium: 455mg | Vitamin A: 25IU | Calcium: 12mg | Iron: 2.9mg

40. Air Fryer Steak Bites & Mushrooms

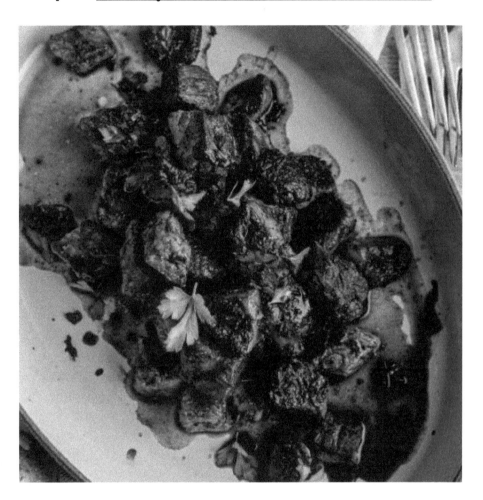

Prep Time: 10 mins

Cook Time: 18 mins

Total Time: 28 mins

Ingredients

- 1 lb. (454 g) steaks, cut into 1/2" cubes (ribeye, sirloin, tri-tip, or what you prefer)
- 8 oz. (227 g) mushrooms (cleaned, washed, and halved)

- 2 tablespoons (30 ml) butter, melted (or olive oil)
- 1 teaspoon (5 ml) worcestershire sauce
- 1/2 teaspoon (2.5 ml) garlic powder, optional
- Flakey salt, to taste
- Fresh cracked black pepper, to taste
- Minced parsley, garnish
- Melted butter, for finishing - optional
- Chili flakes, for finishing - optional
- **Instructions**
- Rinse and thoroughly pat dry the steak cubes. Combine the steak cubes and mushrooms. Coat with the melted butter and then season with Worcestershire sauce, optional garlic powder, and a generous seasoning of salt and pepper.
- Preheat the Air Fryer at 400°F for 4 minutes.
- Spread the steak and mushrooms in an even layer in the air fryer basket. Air fry at 400°F for 10-18 minutes, shaking and flipping and the steak and mushrooms 2 times through the cooking process (time depends on your preferred doneness, the thickness of the steak, size of air fryer).
- Check the steak to see how well done it is cooked. If you want the steak more done, add an extra 2-5 minutes of cooking time.
- Garnish with parsley and drizzle with optional melted butter and/or optional chili flakes. Season with additional salt & pepper if desired. Serve warm.

Nutrition Facts

Calories: 401kcal | Carbohydrates: 3g | Protein: 32g | Fat: 29g | Saturated Fat: 14g | Cholesterol: 112mg | Sodium: 168mg | Potassium: 661mg | Sugar: 1g | Vitamin A: 255IU | Vitamin C: 1.6mg | Calcium: 11mg | Iron: 3.1mg

41.   Air fryer Steak Tips

Prep Time: 5 minutes

Cook Time: 9 minutes

Total Time: 14 minutes

Servings: 3

Ingredients

- 1.5 lb steak or beef chuck for a cheaper version cut to 3/4 inch cubes
- Air Fryer Steak Marinade
- 1 tsp oil
- 1/4 tsp salt
- 1/2 tsp black pepper, freshly ground
- 1/2 tsp dried garlic powder
- 1/2 tsp dried onion powder
- 1 tsp Montreal Steak Seasoning
- 1/8 tsp cayenne pepper
- Air Fryer Asparagus
- 1 lb Asparagus, tough ends trimmed (could replace with spears of zucchini)
- 1/4 tsp salt
- 1/2 tsp oil (optional)

Instructions

- Preheat the air fryer at 400F for about 5 minutes.
- Meanwhile, trim the steak of any fat and cut it into cubes. Then, toss with the ingredients for the marinade (oil, salt, black pepper, Montreal seasoning, onion and garlic powder & the cayenne pepper) and massage the spices into the meat to coat evenly. Do this in a ziplock bag for easier cleanup.
- Spray the bottom of the air fryer basket with nonstick spray if you have any and spread the prepared meat along the bottom of it. Cook the beef steak tips for about 4-6 minutes and check for doneness.
- Toss the asparagus with 1/2 tsp oil and 1/4 tsp salt until evenly

coated.

- Once the steak bites are browned to your liking, toss them around and move to one side. Add the asparagus to the other side of the air fryer basket and cook for another 3 minutes.
- Remove the steak tips and the asparagus to a serving plate and serve while hot.

Nutrition Facts

- Calories: 526| |Fat: 34g|Saturated Fat: 14g|Cholesterol:138mg|Sodium: 703mg|Potassium:913mg|Carbohydrates:6g|Fiber:3g|Sugar:2g|Protein: 49g|Calcium: 52mg|Iron: 7.1mg

42. Easy Air Fryer Steak Bites

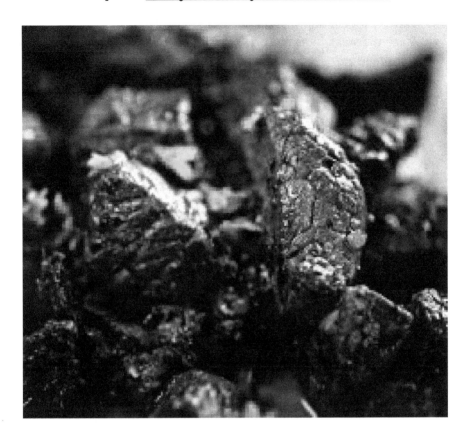

Prep Time: 5 minutes

Cook Time: 9 minutes

Total Time: 14 minutes

Yield: 2-4 servings

Ingredients

- Sirloin Steak Bites or a 1lb. sirloin steak cut into bite-size pieces
- Steak seasoning or salt and pepper
- Olive oil

Instructions

- Start by preheating your air fryer to 390° or 400°.
- Place the steak bites in a bowl and add about a tablespoon of steak seasoning or season with salt and pepper.
- Pour in a tablespoon of olive oil and toss to coat all of the steak bites.
- Place the steak bites in a single layer in your air fryer basket and cook for 5 minutes.
- Turn the steak bites over and cook for an additional 4 minutes for a medium steak. Cook for an additional 2-3 minutes for medium-well and a couple of minutes less for medium-rare.
- Remove from the air fryer and allow them to rest for 5-10 minutes so the meat will retain its juices.
- Enjoy a salad or with your favorite veggies for lunch or dinner!

Nutritional Value

- Calories: 572kcal | Carbohydrates: 1g | Protein: 46g | Fat: 43g | Saturated Fat: 22g | Cholesterol: 168mg | Sodium: 219mg | Potassium: 606mg | Sugar: 1g | Calcium: 16mg | Iron: 4mg

43. Air Fryer Steak Bites (With Or Without Potatoes)

Prep Time: 10 mins

Cook Time: 20 mins

Total Time: 30 mins

Servings: 4 Servings

Ingredients

- 1 lb. (454 g) steaks, cut into 1/2" cubes & patted dry
- 1/2 lb. (227 g) potatoes (optional), cut into 1/2" pieces
- 2 tablespoons (30 ml) butter, melted (or oil)
- 1 teaspoon (5 ml) worcestershire sauce
- 1/2 teaspoon (2.5 ml) garlic powder
- Salt, to taste
- Black pepper, to taste
- Minced parsley, garnish
- Melted butter for finishing, optional
- Chili flakes, for finishing, optional

Instructions

- Heat a large pot of water to a boil and then add the potatoes. Cook for about 5 minutes, or until nearly tender, and then drain.
- Combine the steak cubes and blanched potatoes. Coat with the melted butter and then season with Worcestershire sauce, garlic powder, salt, and pepper.
- Preheat the Air Fryer at 400°F for 4 minutes.
- Spread the steak and potatoes in an even layer in an air fryer basket. Air fry at 400°F for 10-18 minutes, shaking and flipping and the steak and potatoes about 3 times through the cooking process (time depends on your preferred doneness, the thickness of the steak, and size of air fryer).
- Check the steak to see how well done it is cooked. If you want the

steak more done, add an extra 2-5 minutes of cooking time.
- Garnish with parsley and drizzle with optional melted butter and/or optional chili flakes. Season with additional salt & pepper if desired. Serve warm

Nutrition

- Calories: 321kcal | Carbohydrates: 8g | Protein: 24g | Fat: 22g | Saturated Fat: 11g | Cholesterol: 84mg | Sodium: 130mg | Potassium: 550mg | Fiber: 1g | Sugar: 1g | Vitamin A: 192IU | Vitamin C: 6mg | Calcium: 25mg | Iron: 4mg

44. Perfect Air Fryer Steak

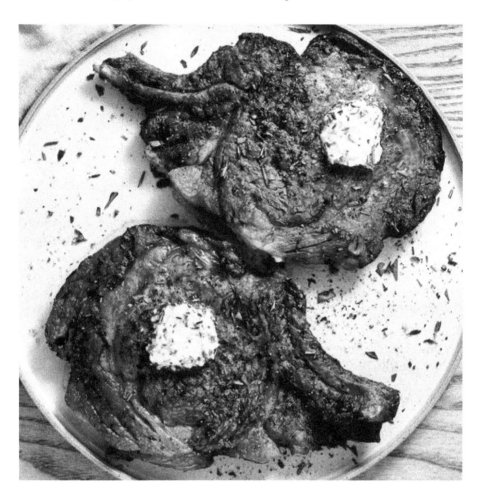

Prep Time: 20 minutes ,Cook Time: 12 minutes ,Resting Time: 5 minutes

Total Time: 32 minutes ,Servings: 2

Ingredients

- 2 8 oz Ribeye steak
- Salt
- Freshly cracked black pepper
- Olive oil

- Garlic Butter
- 1 stick unsalted butter softened
- 2 tbsp fresh parsley chopped
- 2 tsp garlic minced
- 1 tsp Worcestershire Sauce
- 1/2 tsp salt

Instructions

- Prepare Garlic Butter by mixing butter, parsley garlic, Worcestershire sauce, and salt until thoroughly combined.
- Place in parchment paper and roll into a log. Refrigerate until ready to use.
- Remove steak from the fridge and allow to sit at room temperature for 20 minutes. Rub a little bit of olive oil on both sides of the steak and season with salt and freshly cracked black pepper.
- Grease your Air Fryer basket by rubbing a little bit of oil on the basket. Preheat Air Fryer to 400 degrees Fahrenheit. Once preheated, place steaks in the air fryer and cook for 12 minutes, flipping halfway through.
- Remove from air fryer and allow to rest for 5 minutes. Top with garlic butter.

Nutrition

- Calories: 683kcal

45. Air Fryer Steak

Prep Time: 5 min

Cook Time: 12 min

Total Time: 12 min

Yield: 2

Ingredients

- 2 (1 in thick) Steaks Rib Eye, or Tri-Tip), 4 to 6 oz each
- Salt and Pepper to taste
- 2 tablespoons of butter (optional)

Instructions

- If your air fryer requires preheating, preheat your air fryer.
- Set the temperature to 400 degrees Fahrenheit.
- Season your steak with salt and pepper on each side.
- Place the steak in your air fryer basket. Do not overlap the steaks.
- **Medium Steak:** Set the time to 12 minutes and flip the steak at 6.
- **Medium Rare:** For a medium-rare steak, cook the steak for 10 minutes and flip it at 5 minutes.

Nutrition

- Calories: 250|Sodium: 60|Fat: 17|Saturated Fat: 7|Carbohydrates: 0|Fiber: 0|Protein: 23

46. Air Fryer Steak

Prep Time: 5 Minutes

Cook Time: 8 Minutes

Rest Time: 5 Minutes

Total Time: 18 Minutes

Servings: 2 Steaks

Ingredients

- 2 steaks 1" thick, ribeye, sirloin, or striploin
- 1 tablespoon olive oil
- 1 tablespoon salted butter melted
- Steak seasoning to taste

Instructions

- Remove steaks from the fridge at least 30 minutes before cooking.
- Preheat air fryer to 400°F.
- Rub the steaks with olive oil and melted butter. Generously season on each side.
- Add the steaks to the air fryer basket and cook for 8-12 minutes (flipping after 4 minutes) or until steaks reach desired doneness.
- Remove steaks from the air fryer and transfer them to a plate. Rest at least 5 minutes before serving.
- Top with additional butter if desired and serve.

Nutrition Information

- Calories: 582, Carbohydrates: 1g, Protein: 46g, Fat: 45g, Saturated Fat: 19g, Cholesterol: 153mg, Sodium: 168mg, Potassium: 606mg, Sugar: 1g, Vitamin A: 209IU, Calcium: 16mg, Iron: 4mg

Vegetables Recipes

47. Nutty Pumpkin with Blue Cheese

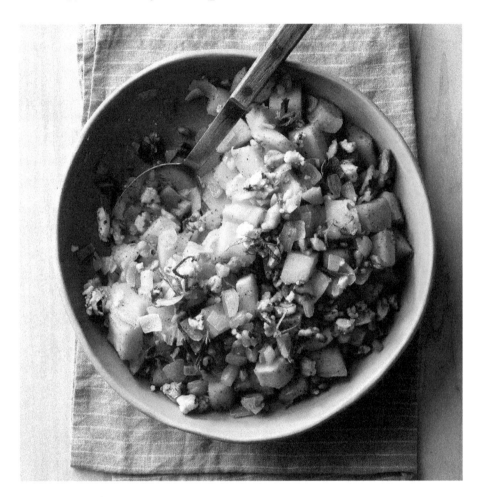

Prep Time :30 minutes

Ingredients:

- ½ small pumpkin
- 2 oz. blue cheese, cubed
- 2 tbsp. pine nuts1 tbsp. olive oil½ cup baby spinach, packed

- 1 spring onion, sliced
- 1 radish, thinly sliced
- 1 tsp. vinegar

Instructions:

- Preheat the air fryer to 330 degrees F.
- Place the pine nuts in a baking dish and toast them for 5 minutes. Set aside. Peel the pumpkin and chop it into small pieces.
- Place in the baking dish and toss with the olive oil. I
- ncrease the temperature to 390 degrees and cook the pumpkin for about 20 minutes.
- Make sure to toss every 5 minutes or so. Place the pumpkin in a serving bowl.
- Add baby spinach, radish and spring onion. Toss with the vinegar.
- Stir in the cubed blue cheese. Top with the toasted pine nuts.

Nutrition Facts

Calories 495, Carbohydrates 29 g, Fat 27 g, Protein 9 g

48. Eggplant Cheeseburger

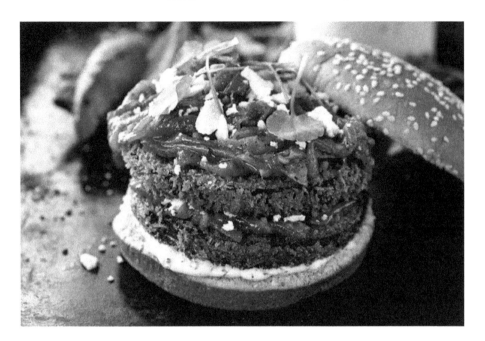

Prep Time: 10 minutes

Ingredients:

- 1 hamburger bun
- 1 2-inch eggplant slice, cut along the round axis
- 1 mozzarella sliceRed onion cut into 3 rings
- 1 lettuce leaf
- ½ tbsp. tomato sauce
- 1 pickle, sliced

Instructions:

- Preheat the air fryer to 330 degrees F.
- Place the eggplant slice and roast for 6 minutes.
- Place the mozzarella slice on top of the eggplant and cook for 30 more seconds.
- Spread the tomato sauce on one half of the bun.
- Place the lettuce leaf on top of the sauce.
- Place the cheesy eggplant on top of the lettuce.

- Top with onion rings and pickles.
- Top with the other bun half and enjoy.

Nutrition Facts

Calories 399, Carbohydrates 21 g, Fat 17 g, Protein 8 g

49. Veggie Meatballs

Prep Time: 30 minutes

Ingredients:

- 2 tbsp. olive oil
- 2 tbsp. soy sauce
- 1 tbsp. flax meal
- 2 cups cooked chickpeas
- ½ cup sweet onion, diced
- ½ cup grated carrots
- ½ cup roasted cashewsJuice of 1 lemon
- ½ tsp. turmeric1 tsp. cumin
- 1 tsp. garlic powder
- 1 cup rolled oats

Instructions:

- Preheat the air fryer to 350 degrees F.
- Combine the oil, onions, and carrots into a baking dish and cook them in the air fryer for 5 minutes.
- Meanwhile, ground the oats and cashews in a food processor. Place them in a large bowl. Process the chickpeas with the lemon juice and soy sauce, until smooth. Add them to the bowl as well.
- Add the onions and carrots to the bowl with the chickpeas.
- Stir in all of the remaining ingredients, and mix until fully incorporated. Make 12 meatballs out of the mixture.
- Increase the temperature to 370 degrees. Cook the meatballs for about 12 minutes..

Nutrition Facts

Calories 288, Carbohydrates 32 g, Fat 21 g, Protein 6 g

50. Crunchy Parmesan Zucchini

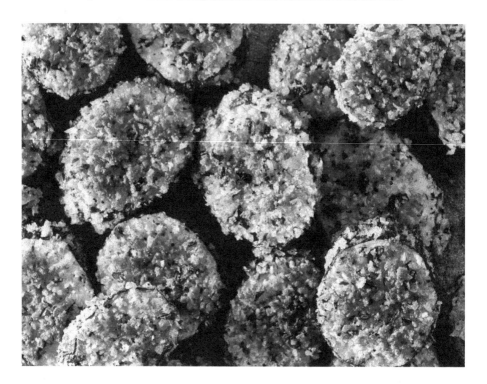

Prep Time: 40 minutes

Ingredients:

- 4 small zucchini cut lengthwise
- ½ cup grated Parmesan cheese
- ½ cup breadcrumbs
- ¼ cup melted butter
- ¼ cup chopped parsley
- 4 garlic cloves, minced
- Salt and pepper, to taste

Instructions:

- Preheat the air fryer to 350 degrees F. In a bowl, mix the breadcrumbs, Parmesan, garlic, and parsley. Season with some salt and pepper, to taste.
- Stir in the melted butter. Arrange the zucchinis with the cut side up.

Spread the mixture onto the zucchini evenly.
- Place half of the zucchinis in your air fryer and cook for 13 minutes.
- Increase the temperature to 370 degrees F and cook for 3 more minutes for extra crunchiness. Repeat with the other batch.

Nutrition Facts

Calories 369, Carbohydrates 14 g, Fat 12 g, Protein 9.5 g

51. Chili Bean Burritos

Prep Time: 30 minutes

Ingredients:

- 6 tortillas
- 1 cup grated cheddar cheese
- 1 can (8 oz.) beans
- 1 tsp. seasoning, by choice

Instructions:

- Preheat the air fryer to 350 degrees F.
- Mix the beans with the seasoning.
- Divide the bean mixture between the tortillas. Top the beans with cheddar cheese.
- Roll the burritos and arrange them on a lined baking dish.
- Place in the air fryer and cook for 5 minutes, or to your liking. Serve as desired (I recommend salsa dipping)

Nutrition Facts

Calories 248, Carbohydrates 25 g, Fat 8.7 g, Protein 9 g

Salad Recipes

52. <u>Air Fryer Healthy Southwestern Salad</u>

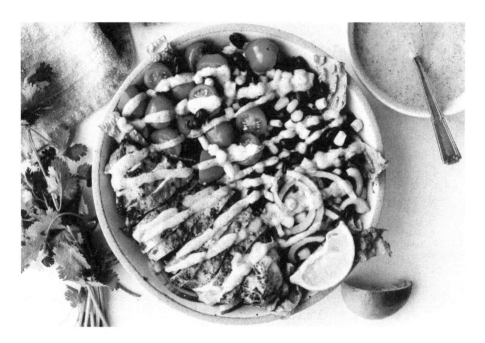

Prep Time: 5 mins

Cook Time: 8 mins

Total Time: 13 mins

Ingredients

Kitchen Gadgets:

- Air Fryer
- Air Fryer Grill Pan
- Salad Bowl
- Southwestern Salad Recipe Ingredients:
- 600 g Chickpeas
- 1 Medium Red Pepper

- 200 g Frozen Sweetcorn
- 2 Celery Sticks
- ¼ Medium Cucumber
- ½ Small Red Onion
- 2 Tbsp Extra Virgin Olive Oil
- 1 Tsp Grainy Mustard
- ¼ Tsp Garlic Powder
- 1 Tsp Basil
- 2 Tsp Mexican Seasoning
- Salt & Pepper

Instructions

- Drain and rinse your chickpeas. Chop your red pepper into bite-size cubes. Load into the air fryer basket with the grill attachment the chickpeas, sweetcorn, and pepper. Sprinkle with Mexican seasoning and salt and pepper and cook for 8 minutes at 180c/360f.
- While the air fryer is in action, prep the rest of your salad. Peel and thinly slice your red onion. Clean and thinly dice your cucumber and celery. Load all three into a salad bowl.
- Mix extra virgin olive oil, basil, grainy mustard, and garlic powder. Pour into your salad bowl and mix.
- When the air fryer beeps, load in the ingredients and mix a little more.
- Serve or store into containers for later.

Nutrition

- Calories: 384kcal | Carbohydrates: 58g | Protein: 16g | Fat: 12g | Saturated Fat: 2g | Sodium: 44mg | Potassium: 737mg | Fiber: 15g | Sugar: 12g | | Vitamin C: 45mg | Calcium: 127mg | Iron: 6mg

53. Kale Salad with Air Fryer Herb Chicken Breast

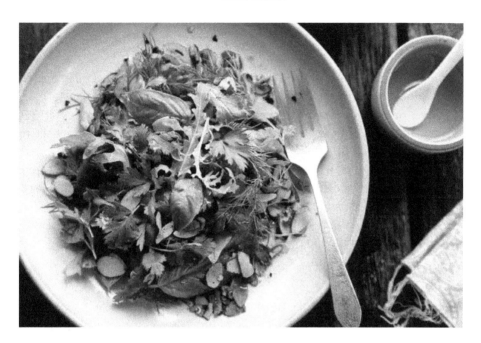

Prep Time: 20 mins

Cook Time: 20 mins

Total Time: 40 mins

Ingredients

- 1 Tablespoon Panko (Bread Crumbs)
- 2 Tablespoons Mixed Dry Herbs Use your favorite blend
- 1 Teaspoon Smoked Paprika
- 1 Teaspoon Salt
- 1 Tablespoon Olive Oil
- 1.5 Pounds Chicken Breast Pounded Evenly
- 1 Cup Corn Kernels From about 2 years, if fresh
- 8 Strawberries, Sliced & Quartered
- 1/2 Ounce Goat Cheese

- 2 Avocados, halved and sliced
- 2 Hard Boiled Eggs, sliced
- 2 Tablespoons Extra Virgin Olive Oil
- 16 Ounce Bag Baby Kale Greens (Washed & Ready)

Instructions

- Combine panko, herbs, smoked paprika, salt, and olive oil in a small bowl to make a paste. Apply this evenly to the chicken breast.
- Cook the chicken in a preheated air fryer for 20 minutes at 370 degrees. Let it rest outside of the air fryer for 5 minutes before slicing for the salad
- In a large salad bowl or serving plate, place your bed of salad greens and then add the corn, strawberries, goat cheese, avocado, hard-boiled eggs, and chicken
- Drizzle the extra virgin olive oil over the top and then season lightly with salt and pepper

Nutrient Value

- Calories: 572kcal | Carbohydrates: 1g | Protein: 46g | Fat: 43g | Saturated Fat: 22g | Cholesterol: 168mg | Sodium: 219mg | Potassium: 606mg | Sugar: 1g | Calcium: 16mg | Iron: 4mg

54. Easy Air Fryer Broccoli

Prep Time: 5 Minutes

Cook Time: 6 Minutes

Total Time: 11 Minutes

Ingredients

- 2 heads of broccoli, cut into bite-sized pieces
- 2 tablespoons olive oil
- Sea salt, to taste
- Fresh cracked black pepper, to taste

Instructions

- 2 heads of broccoli, cut into bite-sized pieces
- 2 tablespoons olive oil
- Sea salt, to taste
- Fresh cracked black pepper, to taste

Nutrition Information

- Calories: 126| Total Fat: 8g| Saturated Fat: 1g| Trans Fat: 0g| Unsaturated Fat: 6g| Cholesterol: 0mg| Sodium: 222mg| Carbohydrates: 14g| Fiber: 6g| Sugar: 3g| Protein: 4g

55. Roasted Vegetable Pasta Salad

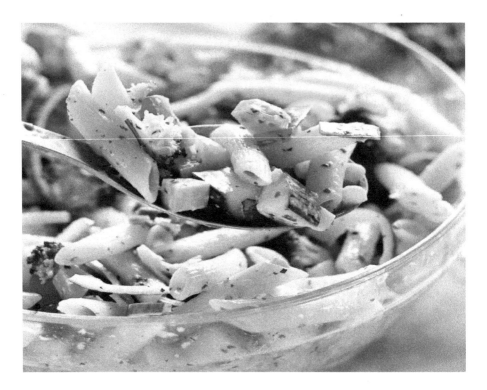

Prep Time: 40 minutes Cook Time: 1 hour 45 minutes Total Time: 2 hours 25 minutes

Ingredients

- 3 eggplant (small)
- 1 tablespoon olive oil
- 3 zucchini (medium-sized. Aka courgette.
- 1 tablespoon olive oil
- 4 tomatoes (medium. Cut in eighths)
- 300 g pasta (large, shaped pasta. 4 cups)
- 2 bell peppers (any color)
- 175 g cherry tomatoes (sliced. Or tomatoes cut into small chunks. 1 cup)
- 2 teaspoons salt (or salt sub)
- 8 tablespoons parmesan cheese (grated)

- 125 ml italian dressing (bottled, fat free/ 1/2 cup / 4 oz)
- Basil (few leaves of fresh)

Instructions

- Wash eggplant, slice off and discard the green end. Do not peel. Slice the eggplant into 1 cm (1/2 inch) thick rounds. If using a paddle-type air fryer such as an Actifry™, put in a pan with 1 tablespoon of olive oil. If using a basket-type such as an AirFryer™, toss with 1 tablespoon of olive oil and put in the basket. Cook for about 40 minutes until quite soft and no raw taste left. Set aside.
- Wash zucchini/courgette, slice off and discard the green end. Do not peel. Slice into 1 cm (1/2 inch) thick rounds. If using a paddle-type air fryer such as an Actifry™, put in a pan with 1 tablespoon of olive oil. If using a basket-type such as an AirFryer™, toss with 1 tablespoon of olive oil and put in the basket. Cook for about 25 minutes until quite soft and no raw taste left. Set aside.
- Wash and chunk the tomatoes. If using an Actifry 2 in 1, arranged in a top grill pan. If using a basket-type air fryer, arrange it in the basket. Spray lightly with cooking spray. Roast for about 30 minutes until reduced in size and starting to brown. Set aside.
- Cook the pasta according to pasta directions, empty into a colander, run cold water over it to wash some starch off, drain, set aside to cool.
- Wash, seed, and chop the bell pepper; put into a large bowl. Wash and slice the cherry tomatoes (or small-chunk the regular tomato); add to that bowl. Add the roast veggies, the pasta, the salt, the dressing, the chopped basil, and the parm, and toss all with your (clean) hands to mix well.
- Set in fridge to chill and marinate.
- Serve chilled or room temperature.

Nutrition

- Serving: 1g | Calories: 121kcal | Carbohydrates: 23g | Protein: 5g | Fat: 4g | Saturated Fat: 1g | Sodium: 417mg | Potassium: 471mg | Fiber: 4g | Sugar: 7g | Vitamin C: 34.2mg | Calcium: 53mg | Iron: 0.8mg

56.   Air Fryer Buffalo Chicken Salad

Prep Time: 15 Mins Cook Time: 15 Mins Total Time: 30 Mins

Ingredients

- 1 pound boneless, skinless chicken breasts, thick sides pounded to make an even thickness
- 1/2 cup WHOLE30 Buffalo Vinaigrette
- 6 cups chopped romaine lettuce
- 1 cup thinly sliced celery
- 1/2 cup shredded carrot
- 3-4 tbsp WHOLE30 Ranch Dressing
- 1 small ripe avocado, peeled, pitted, and sliced
- 1 cup cherry tomatoes, halved
- Freshly ground black pepper
- 2 tsp finely chopped chives

Instructions

- IN a large resealable plastic bag, combine chicken and WHOLE30 Buffalo Vinaigrette. Massage to coat. Seal bag and marinate in the refrigerator for at least 2 hours and up to 4 hours.
- PREHEAT air fryer* to 375°F. Remove chicken from bag; discard marinade. Add the chicken to the air fryer. Cook until chicken is no longer pink and the internal temperature is 170°F, turning once about 15 minutes. Let stand while making the salad.
- IN a large bowl, combine the romaine, celery, and carrot. Add the WHOLE30 Ranch Dressing; toss to combine. Divide salad among four serving plates.
- SLICE the chicken. Top the salads with sliced chicken, avocado, and cherry tomatoes. Season to taste with black pepper. Sprinkle with chives.

Nutrients Value

- Calories: 122| Fat: 8g| Sat fat: 2g| Unsatfat: 5g| Protein: 10g| Carbohydrate| 0g Fiber 0g| Sugars 0g| Added sugars: 0g| Sodium: 254mg

57. Cajun Potato Salad Recipe

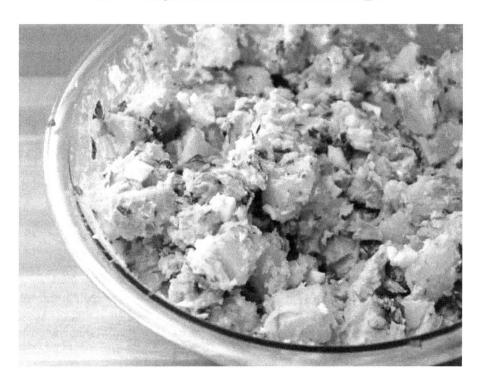

Prep Time: 10 Minutes

Cook Time: 20 Minutes

Total Time: 30 Minutes

Ingredients

- 2 1/2 lb red potatoes, quartered
- 2 tablespoons avocado oil (or grapeseed, coconut, or vegetable)
- 3 tablespoons The Fit Cook Southern Creole
- pinch of sea salt & pepper
- 2 slices cooked bacon, chopped and crumbled

Salad Sauce

- 2/3 cup light mayo (I used olive oil mayo)

105

- 7oz 2% Greek yogurt
- 1/8 cup Dijon mustard (or more to taste)
- 5 BOILED eggs, chopped
- 1 cup diced Dill pickles (OR sweet if you prefer)
- 1/2 medium red onion, diced
- Sea salt & pepper to taste

Steps

- Set the air-fryer to 400F (or oven to 420F).
- In a large bowl, toss the sliced potatoes with oil and seasoning. Add the potatoes to the air-fryer basket. Air-fry for about 20 minutes, or until the potatoes are cooked through and the edges are crispy.
- Air-fried Cajun Potato Salad
- Mix the ingredients for the sauce.
- Cook up some bacon in a skillet until crispy.
- Allow the pieces to cool on a paper towel, then chop into pieces.
- Once the potatoes have finished air-frying, LIGHTLY mash about 40-50% of the potatoes in a bowl, then fold in the remaining potatoes and mix. Add the sauce and the remaining ingredients and fold everything together.
- Season to taste using salt & pepper, dill (or sweet) pickles, mustard, or Greek yogurt. Cover with plastic and store in the fridge for at least 20 minutes, but it's much better overnight.

Nutrient Value

- Calories: 491
- Protein: 20g
- Fat: 16g
- Carbs: 72g
- Fiber: 5g
- Sugar: 9g

58. Air Fryer Squash With Kale Salad

Prep Time: 5 minutes

Cook Time: 10 minutes

Total Time: 15 minutes

Ingredients

- Squash
- 1 medium delicata squash (see note 1)
- Salt and pepper to taste (or other spices)
- Salad
- 8 oz kale or other green, chopped
- 1 cup grape or cherry tomatoes, halved
- 2 cups cucumber, sliced
- 1/2 cup pomegranate seeds
- 1/4 cup squash seeds, roasted, optional
- 1/2 avocado, sliced, optional
- 1/2 cup vegan honey mustard dressing, or any dressing

Instructions

Cut The Squash: If using delicata, cut the top and bottom off, then slice it lengthwise down the middle. Cut the delicata (or other squash) into half-inch thick pieces. You can leave delicate in a half-ring shape, or you can slice it into smaller pieces (especially if feeding littles) (bigger is fine, but will take longer to cook). If you find the squash hard to cut, try microwaving it for a minute or two first.

Save The Seeds: I highly recommend saving the seeds and roasting them! It's so easy, and worth it. I find it easiest to scoop out the seeds and membrane with a grapefruit spoon. Then fill a medium-sized bowl with water, so that the seeds mostly float to the top as I free them from the membrane.

Season: Lightly spray the squash with water, (or oil, if that's your thing) and season with salt, pepper, and whatever else you like (sometimes I use garlic, chili, etc.)

Air Fryer Method: Add to your air fryer. They will get crispier if they are in a single layer. Air fry at 375 degrees F (or 191 degrees C) for about 10 minutes, shaking halfway through. If you like it more browned, you can keep cooking for another 5 minutes or so.

Oven Method: Line a baking tray with a silicone baking mat or parchment paper. Lay the squash pieces out in a single layer with a little breathing room (about an inch) between each piece. Bake at 400 degrees Fahrenheit (or 205 degrees Celsius) for about 20-25 minutes, flipping the pieces halfway through.

Store: Refrigerate leftovers in an airtight container. The salad will keep for about 3 days (if dressed), the squash about 5 days (keep separate from the salad if possible). The seeds should keep on the counter in an airtight container for about 5 days.

Nutrients Value

- Calories: 213
- Total Fat: 5.2g
- Sodium: 419.8mg
- Sugar: 23.6g
- Carbohydrates: 37.1mg
- Protein:7.1g
- Vitamin C: 165.5mg

59. Fried Chickpeas In The Air Fryer

Prep Time: 2 minutes

Cook Time: 12 minutes

Total Time: 14 minutes

Ingredients

- 1 1/2 cups chickpeas 1 15 ounces can drain & rinse
- Spritz cooking spray
- 2 teaspoons **Nutrition Facts**al yeast flakes
- 1/2 teaspoon granulated onion
- Pinch salt

Instructions

- Put the drained chickpeas into the air fryer basket. Set the air fryer for 400 degrees and 12 minutes.
- Cook the plain chickpeas for the first 5 minutes. This will dry them out.
- Then open the basket, spritz the chickpeas with oil, give a shake, and spritz them again. Sprinkle on **Nutrition Facts**al yeast flakes, granulated onion, and a pinch of salt.
- Return the basket to the air fryer and cook for the remaining 7 minutes.
- Test a chickpea to see if it's done enough for you. Depending on your air fryer, the softness of your chickpeas, and your personal preferences, you may want to cook them for an additional 3 to 5 minutes. If desired, add another pinch of salt before serving.

Nutrition

- Calories: 105kcal | Carbohydrates: 17g | Protein: 5g | Fat: 1g | Sodium: 4mg | Potassium: 198mg | Fiber: 4g | Sugar: 2g | Vitamin A: 15IU | Vitamin C: 0.8mg | Calcium: 30mg | Iron: 1.8mg

60. Air Fryer Buffalo Chicken Tenders Salad

Prep Time: 15 minutes Cook Time: 25 minutes Total Time: 40 minutes

Ingredients

Chicken Tenders:

- ½ cup blanched almond flour
- 1 tsp sea salt
- 1 tsp paprika
- ¼ tsp ground black pepper
- 2 large chicken breasts, sliced lengthwise into ½" strips
- ¼ cup tapioca flour
- 2 tbsp garlic-infused olive oil
- Avocado oil cooking spray

Salad:

- 2 hearts of romaine, chopped
- 1 cup carrots, coarsely-shredded
- 1 cup grape tomatoes, halved
- 1 bunch scallions, green tops only, chopped
- 1 red pepper, diced
- Your other favorite salad ingredients

Ranch Dressing:

- ½ Batch of my dairy-free homemade ranch dressing recipe (paleo, whole30, low fodmap)

Buffalo Sauce:

- ⅓ cup Paleo Low-FODMAP hot sauce
- 3 tbsp ghee, melted
- 1 tbsp garlic-infused olive oil
- ½ tbsp coconut aminos

Instructions

- Preheat the air fryer to 370° F for 10 minutes. While your air fryer preheats, combine almond flour, sea salt, paprika, and pepper in a large bowl, whisk to combine, and set aside. Place chicken strips in another large bowl. Add tapioca flour to the bowl and toss with your hands to coat the strips evenly. Add the garlic-infused oil and toss again to coat. Dredge each strip in the almond flour mixture, shaking off the excess, and set on a plate.
- Once your air fryer has preheated, spray the pan with cooking spray. Using tongs, place half of the breaded chicken strips in the pan in one layer, ideally not touching one another. Spray the strips lightly with cooking spray. Air fry for 12 minutes, flipping halfway through. Once the first batch has cooked, place it on a clean plate using a clean set of tongs and set aside. Using tongs, take one of the thickest strips out of the air fryer and check its temperature using an instant-read thermometer. The temperature of cooked chicken should be at least 165° F (75° C) to be safely consumed. Once the first batch is at the proper temperature, repeat these steps for the second half of the strips.
- While the chicken strips are frying, prepare a half-batch of my dairy-free homemade ranch dressing recipe, cover, and refrigerate until ready to serve. Chop the ingredients under "salad," place in a large serving bowl, and refrigerate.
- A minute or two before the chicken strips are done, in a large bowl, add the ingredients under "buffalo sauce," whisk to combine, and set aside until all the chicken strips are cooked. If the sauce solidifies, microwave it (covered) for about 20 seconds and whisk again.
- Once the second batch of strips has finished cooking, if desired, place the first batch back in the air fryer on top of the second batch and air fry at 370° F for a minute or so until heated (I typically skip this step as they're going on a cold salad anyway). Using tongs, take each strip out of the air fryer, dip in the buffalo sauce until fully-coated, and place it on a plate. Chop strips horizontally into small pieces if desired and serve on top of the salad with the ranch dressing.

Nutrient Value

- Total Fat: 30.8gg Sodium: 1321.9mg Sugar: 6.7g Vitamin A: 567.5ug
- Carbohydrates: 21.4g Protein:29.8g Vitamin C: 56.8mg

CPSIA information can be obtained
at www.ICGtesting.com
Printed in the USA
LVHW081945110621
689903LV00002B/190